Diets Don't Work

Diets Don't Work

by Bob Schwartz

Breakthru Publishing, Galveston, Texas

COPYRIGHT © 1982 BY ROBERT M. SCHWARTZ

ISBN 0-942540-00-X

LIBRARY OF CONGRESS
CATALOG CARD NO.: 82-70262

Published by
BREAKTHRU PUBLISHING
1509 Broadway
Galveston, TX 77550

Printed in the United States of America

ACKNOWLEDGMENTS

To Werner Erhard: Whose training led me to my breakthrough and who, by his example, gave me the courage to share it with the world.

To Cherie Carter-Scott: Who taught me to see that people have their own answers and to trust myself and go for my dreams.

To Alan Doelit: A pioneer who, in 1971, took sensory awareness into the realm of weight loss and started to discover the truth about diets.

To Kate Solovieff Martin, Maria Demetriou, Jerry and Kathy Matacio, Carol Costello, and Carmen Keltner, who helped me put the pieces together.

To the 1,000 who went through the Diets Don't Work seminars.

And to the love of my life, Leah: for losing her 40 lbs. and always making me right.

Some of the names in this book have been changed, but the facts are accurate.

Again, I want to thank you if you were one of the more than 1,000 people to go through the Diets Don't Work Seminar. You made this book possible.

PREFACE

Everyone who takes the Diets Don't Work Seminar has a different experience of the seminar and of themselves. That is what is meant to happen. Each person has a unique relationship to his or her weight problem. The purpose of the seminar is to discover exactly what that relationship is and to transform it so that weight is ended as a problem forever.

In this book, Bob Schwartz recreates the experience of actually being in the seminar and going through the same process that people go through in the seminar room. He takes you step by step through the discovery of how the weight got there in the first place and how to take it off without effort or dieting. It involves a transformation not only of your body, but of your entire attitude toward yourself and your life.

This book is intended to let you do four things:

• Discover the real reasons you have not lost weight and kept it off;

• Learn a method for losing weight without dieting;

• Develop a new relationship with yourself, a new self-image based on being a naturally thin person;

• End weight as a problem in your life forever.

Congratulations. By picking up this book, you've taken the first step toward living the rest of your life as a naturally thin person.

The Editors

TABLE OF CONTENTS

Don't Try — Do!
Do It Passionately
The Only Real Change Comes From Within

Part I:
The Awful Truth About Dieting:
What You Suspected Is True!

CHAPTER 1

Diets Don't Work

A 99.5% Failure Rate

I've lost over 2,000 pounds and spent twenty-four years in my health spas helping thousands of people lose weight. In the process I've discovered something you probably suspected all along — *diets don't work.*

I've discovered something else, too. Not only don't diets work, they're actually designed to *fail.* It's not you or your lack of will power that's the problem. It's that diets by their very nature simply don't work.

Do you know how many people actually get the results they want by dieting? One out of every 200! The failure rate of diets and weight-loss programs is 99.5%

The Washington Post reports that out of every 200 people who go on a diet, only ten lose all the weight they set out to lose.* And of those ten, only one keeps it off for any reasonable length of time. *In*

---

* Special to *The Washington Post* by Arthur Frank.
Reprinted in *The Houston Chronicle,* December 8, 1980.

other words, only one person out of every 200 loses all their excess weight and keeps it off by dieting.

Not only that, but in studying that one person I discovered that they do *everything* compulsively. They even brush their teeth and clean their home compulsively. They find diets easy. They ate compulsively and now they diet compulsively. If necessary, they'd eat hardboiled eggs and grapefruit today and every day till doomsday. If being compulsive is a prerequisite for having diets work, then most of us aren't going to have much success.

Beware! Treacherous Waters

Let me ask you a question. Suppose you're standing on the bank of a river, and the river is filled with man-eating sharks. The sharks are so angry and hungry that the water is churning and boiling over the sides of the banks. On the other side of the river is Happyland, where all the thin people live. If only you can get to the other side, you will have exactly the body you want to have, but you have to cross the river first.

There are 200 people ahead of you, and they all jump into the river and start swimming to Happyland. Immediately the sharks attack, the water churns even more violently, and finally only one of the 200 pulls himself up onto the other bank. He waves at you and calls across the river, "Hey, come on over. It's great over here!"

Your group of 200 is next. Would you go? Probably not. You might yell back, "I'm going to wait till Monday," or "I'll hold off till my next New Year's resolution." Is it any wonder we approach diets with something less than enthusiasm? You'd have to be crazy to jump into that water. But we do. *Over and over again.*

Diets Do Work — In Reverse

At my health spas we have one of the most successful weight-*gain* programs in the country, based on exactly the same principles people have been using to *lose* weight. Say a person has been trying for years, but no matter how much they eat, no matter how much they exercise, no matter how many calories they stuff into their mouth, they can't gain weight.

What we do with them always works. We put them on a diet. A

weight *loss* diet. It doesn't matter what kind — high carbohydrate, high protein, high fat — just as long as it's a diet intended to make them lose weight.

We put them on this diet for three days. Most of them have a terrible time because they've never dieted and are horrified at the thought of losing more weight. If they stick to the diet for three days, they may lose anywhere from two to seven pounds. At this point their confidence in our expertise hits rock bottom, but then we take them off the diet and allow them to eat normally. Within a few days they've gained all the weight back — *plus some.*

Soon their weight levels off, and immediately we put them back on the same diet for another three days. This time they lose maybe one to five pounds. They're not as scared this time, because they're beginning to understand. We take them off the diet, and again they gain back the weight they lost, plus some.

Again we put them on the same diet for three more days, and this time they *don't lose any weight at all.* And when we take them off, they gain. We keep doing this — one step backward, two steps forward — until they're the weight they want to be.

Sound familiar? Sound like your life? You see, diets do work — in reverse. They're the best method for gaining weight ever discovered.

Sometimes a strange thing happens to these formerly skinny people. We warn them before they start that once we get them going, they may not be able to stop the weight-gain process. They laugh and say they'll cross that bridge when they come to it. When they come to it, it's not so funny.

Why Diets Don't Work: The Diet Mentality

It's starting to sound even worse then you thought, isn't it? Well, you're right. Dieting to lose weight is akin to throwing gasoline on a fire to put it out. Dieting not only doesn't solve the problem, it makes it worse by producing what I call the *Diet Mentality.*

The Diet Mentality has come about because there is agreement in our society that the only way to lose weight is by dieting. But dieting produces absolutely no permanent, positive results. In fact, it makes you feel worse about yourself and probably does more damage than good to your health.

There are five elements to the Diet Mentality:

1. FAT IS BAD. The Diet Mentality is based on the assumption that fat is bad and thin is good. You begin dieting to become thin and good, only to set in motion an endless cycle of dieting and failure.

2. THE VICIOUS CIRCLE OF FAILURE. When I ask people in my seminars to tell me what their experience with dieting has been, they generally slump in their chairs, looking discouraged and beaten. I've heard thousands of people tell the same story. They go on a diet to lose weight. At best they have only partial success before they quit dieting, and then they gain the weight back. They get angry at themselves, feel guilty or ashamed because they failed, go on another diet, and the cycle is repeated.

They start to think of themselves as failures. They don't dare stop dieting, though, because if it's this bad while they're dieting, think how awful it would be if they stopped! The anxiety becomes so intense that they find themselves overeating or going on a binge to cope with it. Most of their time is spent worrying about what they're eating, what they're not eating, how their clothes look, how many pounds they might or might not lose that day, how many calories are in this or that food, and how they should probably exercise more. After a while every thought begins to relate in some way to their weight — and the whole process is a negative one.

No matter how motivated they become, how strict they are on themselves, how hard they try, the outcome is always the same — failure. The trouble with this kind of failure is that in our culture people take it personally. They use it to deflate their self-esteem and self-respect and to beat themselves up. It's very difficult to succeed at anything, especially dieting, with such a poor self-image.

3. DEPRIVATION AND RESTRICTION. Another key element to the Diet Mentality is the mechanism of self-deprivation that it sets up in people's minds. The deprivation comes from not having the foods they want to eat, or the life they want to lead. They have probably already restricted their activities because they're fat — for example, they don't go to the beach, they don't apply for the job they really want, they don't participate in sports, they avoid social gatherings. Constant dieting only adds to those restrictions. It isolates people further from the mainstream of life. Now they can't go on a picnic or to parties or out to lunch with their

co-workers, can't have popcorn at the movies or birthday cake at the office. They've felt left out and deprived because they're fat, and now they feel even more restricted because they're on a diet as well. It's like closing off the rooms of a house one by one until only one room is left, a small, cramped space that feels like a prison.

Over time this kind of deprivation and isolation can only add another negative dimension to the Diet Mentality, sapping all the vitality out of life. It's crazy to think this stifling state of mind could produce positive results. No wonder people have to psyche themselves up for a diet.

4. MISPLACED RESPONSIBILITY. The fourth element of the Diet Mentality is that it gives you the illusion that you're no longer responsible for a basic human function — eating. When you go on Dr. X's Famous Diet, you give up your power to choose when, what, and how much you're going to eat. It carries with it the infuriating feeling that you're one year old again and someone else is in control of what goes in your mouth. And it gives you someone else to blame for your weight problem — Dr. X's Famous Diet didn't work.

When you go off the diet, you come away with the attitude that you can't be trusted with food. Now Sara Lee and Baskin-Robbins are *doing it to you.* If you can give your power away to Dr. X, you can now just as easily give it away to Sara Lee; it's just the flip side of the same coin. Every time you go on a diet and then go on a binge, you reinforce the pattern of placing the responsibility elsewhere. It's a pattern which denies a basic truth: *you* are responsible for what goes into your mouth. How can you ever hope to solve a problem if you believe that someone else is responsible? You're defeated before you start. Obviously, you have no control over anyone other than yourself, and only when you're clear about who is responsible for your weight will you have the power to master it. The Diet Mentality denies you this choice.

5. TREATING THE SYMPTOMS RATHER THAN THE CAUSE. The first two elements of the Diet Mentality might perhaps be turned around with positive thinking. But the fifth element is the bottom-line reason why diets don't work and never will.

Technically it's true that people gain weight because they put more food in their bodies than their bodies can use, and their bodies store the excess as fat. On the surface this looks like the cause for overweight, and so dieting seems like a perfectly reasonable solution.

What dieting can never do is bring to light the things that cause people to put more food into their bodies than their bodies need in the first place. This, rather than the activity of overeating, is truly the source of the problem. What stimulates people to overeat? In my seminars I've found that the cause is unique to each person. And until that cause is brought to the surface, examined, and dealt with, the pounds will keep coming back no matter how many diets a person goes on.

The Diet Mentality is not a pleasant subject to think about. We've all lived it to some degree, and we know the self-defeating feelings that accompany it. If you're feeling hopeless right now, you're right — it *is* hopeless. Diets will never work. You, however, are not hopeless. You've just been using a method that doesn't work and then blaming yourself for your lack of results. Before we go on, however, I want you to be very clear about your own experience with the Diet Mentality. The following exercise is designed to do this.

EXERCISES (5 minutes)

Write down, as fully and specifically as you can, the answers to the following questions. Take some time to think about your answers, and elaborate as much as possible.

Note: Don't hesitate to write in this book. As your personal workbook, it's meant to be written in. It's yours and yours alone, a journal of your progress toward becoming a thin person. I can't stress enough how important it is to do each and every exercise as you come to it. This book is specifically designed to recreate the experience of the Diets Don't Work Seminar and takes you through a step-by-step process of discovery and revelation. Only when you are truly willing to look at yourself, to get specific, and to take the time and energy to do each exercise are you ready to find your answers.

1. Have diets worked for you in the past?

2. What has happened before when you've gone on a diet?

3. Where is the problem, with you or with the diets you've tried?

4. Do you have any lingering doubts that diets don't work? If so, list what they are:

a.

b.

c.

d.

e.

If you come up with doubts like, "Maybe someday they'll find a better diet," or "Maybe someday I'll get more will power," then ask yourself if you really believe that, and if you're willing to wait that long.

5. What has been your own experience with the Diet Mentality? Write short descriptions of all the times you've gotten hooked into it, and tell how you felt before, during, and after the diet.

Thank you for taking the time and energy to do these exercises. It will put you ahead of the game as we go on. Each time you're

willing to examine yourself and be honest about your relationship
with your weight, you make more progress toward becoming a thin
person.

You Can't Get There From Here

The Diet Mentality can only make you less happy and more fat.
But it is persistent. Most people still insist that it's the only way to
lose weight, even though it's only worked for a very few people.
They keep saying, "All you have to do is eat less and exercise more,
and if you can't do that, it's your own fault you're fat."

Now that you've taken a comprehensive look at what you're
doing when you operate according to the Diet Mentality, you can
begin to see how the Diet Mentality might keep you stuck in a
downward spiral. It's as if all you wanted to do was to go to the
house across the street, but you kept going out to the airport to get
there. Planes don't fly to the house across the street. "You can't get
there from here."

You've probably heard the cliche, "Success breeds success."
Many books have been written on the subject of motivation, and
they've all come to one conclusion: you cannot motivate people
with negativity and failure. You have to build on successes and
positive results.

The Diet Mentality is overwhelmingly negative, self-deflating,
and stifling. We've turned this problem into a punishing ordeal that
never produces the results we want. Even worse, it strips us of our
dignity and mastery over our bodies by implying that we are weak
or defective because we can't make diets work.

Nobody Has the Answer
(And They Don't Want You to Find Out)

No one has an answer to the problem of how to lose weight.
Doctors don't have it. Diet experts don't have it. Psychologists
don't have it. Ministers and clergymen don't have it. Gurus don't
have it. If anyone had it, there would be no more fat people.

Maybe the reason no one has it is that no one's willing to come
out and admit that diets don't work, even though it seems like the
most obvious thing in the world.

Suppose you went to a strange planet, and every time someone
broke their leg, they were given an aspirin and told to go jogging.

As soon as they started hobbling around the track, they fell down and got worse. It would be pretty obvious to you that what was being prescribed for them wasn't working, wouldn't it? Why, then, do you suppose the people on that planet weren't able to see that and change it?

Maybe someone owned an aspirin business. Or a jogging track. And even with the staggering evidence against the aspirin-jogging cure, they didn't want to admit the cure didn't work. There is such a thing as the diet industry, and it may be that there are lots of doctors, diet experts, and psychologists who are wondering what they'd do with their time if someone let out the secret that diets don't work.

Maybe the reasons are more innocent. It's awfully hard to admit you're wrong, especially if you have a lot invested in being right. You don't have to have invested money. You may have invested time, energy, belief, or hope. I'd invested twenty years in diets and exercise, plus my relationships with the thousands of people I'd worked with. It wasn't easy to admit that what I'd been doing didn't work.

I knew a lot of things. I knew about calories — how to accumulate them and how to burn them off. I was an expert on every diet that had come along for twenty years. I knew a lot about the psychology of motivation and weight-loss. But the simple truth is that *what I knew wasn't enough. It didn't work. It was the wrong kind of information.* Forget the investment of time and money; it was my pride that really hurt.

No one wants to be proven wrong. Sometimes we would rather be right and fat than wrong and thin.

While I was writing this book, an incident happened that was a perfect illustration of what I've been talking about. I was coming over the Bay Bridge during rush hour one morning with Kathy, one of my seminar leaders, and she got into a lane that I don't usually use. I asked Kathy why she had chosen that lane, and she said, "This is the best lane. It's the one I always take." Noticing that cars were passing us on both sides and that our lane was moving more slowly than any of the others, I pointed to a blue truck one lane over and said to Kathy, "See that truck? I want you to race it across the bridge, but stay in this lane."

The blue truck started to edge out in front of us, but Kathy was still defending the lane she'd chosen. As he got farther and farther ahead, however, and finally disappeared out of sight, it became harder and harder for her to hold on to her point of view. You see, she was confronted with specific, tangible evidence that what she'd done hadn't worked.

Kathy laughed and admitted that she'd chosen the wrong lane, but a lot of people wouldn't do that. They would keep insisting that they were right, even in the face of overwhelming evidence. That's exactly what's happened with diets.

Beginning the Search for Your Own Answers

As I've said before, I've found through my seminars that everyone has a unique situation with regard to their weight. This is still another reason why the shotgun approach to diets will never work. Each person needs to find their own personal insights and discoveries that will reveal their individual solution to their particular problem.

Before you can reach any goal, it's a good idea to start with where you are right now. The following exercises will help you to have the specific insights that you'll need as we go through this book. Whatever you do, don't use any of the information you gather as a stick to beat yourself with. This is a fact-finding mission only. Your purpose is simply to tell the truth about where you are now and how you feel about it. Please take the time to do the exercises carefully and experience what you feel as you're doing them.

EXERCISES (10 minutes)

1. "My present weight is _____. I wear size_____ pants and size _____ dress or coat. My measurements are:_____(hips), _____(waist),_____(abdomen),_____(upper part of right arm),_____(upper part of right thigh)."

2. Now stand in front of a mirror and say the following sentence out loud, as if you were announcing it to the world and giving away a secret. Keep breathing while you do it:

"I,____(your name)___ , weigh _____ pounds and wear size _____ pants (or dress)."

3. What did you notice about yourself while you were doing exercise 2? What did you hear in your voice? How did you feel when you were saying it?

4. Now stand in front of a mirror and say the same sentence again. This time say it as if you were the one who made your body that way, and it was exactly the way you wanted it to be up to now. Say it as if you'd done it all by yourself and for a very good reason.

5. Complete the following sentence, being as specific and thorough as you can: "I've wanted to lose weight since..."

6. "This is how I feel about being overweight:"

a.

b.

c.

d.

e.

7. "These are the ways I've tried to lose weight in the past:"

a.

b.

c.

d.

e.

8. "These are some of the good reasons I've wanted to lose weight in the past:"

a.

b.

c.

d.

e.

9. "Right now, without knowing any more than I do, these are some of the things I think I should do to lose weight:"

a.

b.

c.

d.

e.

f.

10. "I think these are the reasons I haven't been successful in the past:"

a.

b.

c.

d.

e.

f.

11. We've talked a lot about the Diet Mentality and the over-whelming evidence that it doesn't work. Why do you think people are still trying it? Why do you think it's still around?

12. Are you honestly willing to give up on diets, even if it means admitting that you've been wrong in the past?

CHAPTER 2

A Breakthrough!

My Own Experience with Fat

Many of the people who have come to our health spas have wanted to lose weight, and we thought the answer was obvious: put them on a diet. For twenty years we used every kind of diet and weight-loss plan imaginable. "It should be simple," we thought. "Just follow the plan and the pounds will roll off." Right? Wrong. Some people lost weight, but very few of them lost as much as they wanted to lose and almost all of them gained it right back.

For twenty years we beat our heads against a brick wall with people who said they wanted to lose weight. They would come to the spa, we would put them on a diet, but as soon as they went off the diet, the pounds would return — plus some.

We were willing to try anything. I remember a doctor who came up with the idea of injecting the urine of pregnant women into people while keeping them on a diet of 500 calories a day. I called the American Medical Association to find out if it was appropriate to recommend the treatment to our spa members. "I wouldn't if I were you," they said. "Any one will lose weight if they eat only 500 calories a day, whether they take shots or not!" The problem was that people couldn't go on eating 500 calories a day forever, and as soon as they stopped, the weight would come back. I wrote the urine-injection folks a letter suggesting that, as long as it didn't matter, why not inject people with the urine of Jack LaLanne? They must not have liked my idea very much; they never wrote back.

About that time I became so frustrated that I decided to test the diets myself, even though I didn't need to lose weight. I wanted to show everyone that it couldn't possibly be as hard as they made it out to be. I went on the diet we were using at the time, and although my body ached as if telling me it didn't like what I was doing to it, within a week I'd lost eleven pounds.

I tried the next few diets that came along, with similar, though not so dramatic, results. Then one day I noticed that my pants felt tight. I'd been going on the diets to prove something, to test them out. But now for the first time, I needed to go on a diet. What had been happening, without my being aware of it, was that each time I went on one of the diets, I would lose weight more slowly, and each time I went off, I would gain it back faster.

As time went on, I found that no matter what kind of diet we tried, the same pattern would emerge. I would follow the diet to the letter and lose, say, ten pounds. But two months later I would have gained it back again — plus some. I'd actually developed a weight problem by testing the diets we were using in our spas.

But I wasn't concerned. I knew that I had only to go back on the first diet I'd tried — after all, on that diet I'd lost eleven pounds in a single week. So I followed it religiously, without deviation, and in the same week also managed to jog twenty miles. At the end of the week, I got on the scale expecting great news, only to discover I'd lost only one pound. The next day I went off the diet and within a few days gained five pounds.

At this point I was getting frustrated. I almost decided to get out of the health spa business and open a chain of Italian restaurants. My whole life was starting to be about my weight: I thought about it, read about it, complained about it, worried about it, made elaborate resolutions about it, and got defensive about it.

I tried to ignore it, hide it, forget it, and accept it. Nothing worked. Worse, no one else really knew what to do, either.

I talked to people who had taken the most extreme measures. They'd had their teeth wired together, taken shots, eaten vitamins and liquid protein, meditated, gotten hypnotized, been fussed over, pleaded with, prayed for, and starved. They'd had staples put into their ears and stomachs, taken behavior modification courses, drunk light beer and diet sodas, eaten diet foods, taken diet pills — and nothing had worked well enough to turn them into thin people.

In desperation I looked around and noticed that a lot of the people I saw jogging were thin. "That must be it," I thought. If you jog, you'll get thin." I even thought about putting on my jogging shoes and starting to jog east. When I reached New York, I reasoned, I would be thin. If it happened along the way — say, in Kansas — I would just get on the next bus home. But in my heart I knew I'd never seriously consider starting on that San Francisco to New York run. No, jogging wasn't the answer I was looking for.

Then one day, as I was driving on the freeway, I saw in a flash exactly what we were doing wrong. We and everyone else had been studying fat people to find out how to make them thin. What we should have been doing was studying thin people to find out what makes them thin! They must know something we don't know; they must do something we don't do.

If you want to be rich, you don't study poor people, you study rich people. If you want to be thin, you don't study fat people, you study thin people. They were the ones with the answers. They were the ones who'd been successful at what we were trying to do. It was so simple I couldn't believe we hadn't thought of it before.

I started from scratch and began my journey into the world of thin. I sought out thin people and studied them. I talked to them, observed them, asked them questions, and sneaked around and watched them when they weren't looking.

I wasn't interested in artificially thin people, the ones who had to struggle to keep themselves that way, the ones who were always using fake salad dressing and living on carrot sticks. I wanted to know about the naturally thin people, the ones who never gave a thought to their weight, who could eat anything they wanted and stay thin without the slightest effort. What did they do that we didn't? What did they know?

It was tough going at first. Thin people didn't seem to know what they did. When asked, they would just shrug or look at me as if I were crazy. They would come up with dumb answers like, "Eat less." Or, "Exercise, I guess." Or, "Push away from the table."

You see, naturally thin people don't think about being thin. As diet veterans you and I can go to a smorgasbord laid out with every kind of delicacy and can probably tell exactly how many calories are in every food on the table. We can compare the pie with the cake, the fish with the meat, the salad with the soup. Some of us even know how many calories are in a single leaf of lettuce or one tablespoon of cottage cheese.

Thin people are ignorant of such things, things we're convinced we need to know to be thin. They don't even know how many calories they burn off by running around the block. And they don't care.

The thins were able to tell me virtually nothing about how they got and stayed that way, but I wasn't about to give up. I kept at it, and finally I found the answer.

The Secret of Thin People

I found out what the thin person's secret is, and it amazed me by its simplicity. These are some of the things I learned.

- For almost everyone, being thin is a natural state.
- It can be as easy and as natural to lose weight as it is to gain it.
- Thin people do *four simple things* that fat people don't, and they never diet.
- There are certain reasons people gain weight, certain reasons they keep it, and specific ways to get and keep it off that work.
- You can get and stay thin naturally, without effort or struggle, and enjoy yourself in the process.

What I discovered wasn't just another list of do's and don't's. It was a *way of thinking about food and about eating* based on a simple, natural principle. If you tune into that principle, to that new way of thinking, feeling, and behaving, then you're on the verge of having your thin body back.

It's not weight that's the real problem — it's the mentality behind it. Get rid of the mentality, and the weight comes off by itself, as quickly and as naturally as it came on. You don't have to give it a second thought.

I know because I did it. And so did the hundreds of people I shared the process with in our Diets Don't Work Seminars. We began to think like thin people, feel like thin people, and behave like thin people. We eat real food now, not diet food, and we use real salad dressing. We now know that if we want Rocky Road ice cream, a thousand carrots sticks won't satisfy us.

We don't have to think about our weight anymore. We feel happier, freer, healthier, and more energetic than we ever have in our lives. There's a joy and rightness about living now, as if we'd discovered some treasure that was there all along. And what we learned about weight has affected every other area of our lives.

That's what I mean by ending weight as a problem forever, and that's the purpose of this book. There's a lot more to it than taking off pounds. There's a way of living that will give you joy and peace and take off pounds in the process. My goal in writing this book is to *end weight as a problem in your life forever,* so that you can go on to do all those things you were going to do *after* you lost weight.

A woman named Susan, from Houston, wrote:

"I never realized how much time I spent thinking about my weight problem. When I first started thinking like a thin person, it was as if my mind went blank. I had to think of something to think about, something to do. I got used to it quickly, though, and started planning my promotion, which I received exactly two months after the seminar. It was like discovering a whole new world. I had all this extra time and energy to live life, to do the things I'd always wanted to do, instead of dwelling on the weight problem again and again."

EXERCISE (2 minutes)

If you woke up tomorrow morning with a new body and were exactly the weight you wanted to be, what three things would you do?

a.

b.

c.

(As you think of more things, continue to add to this list. Begin to look forward to the day when these dreams turn into reality.)

CHAPTER 3

Ending Weight As a Problem Forever

The Challenge

You and I are standing right now at a fork in the road. We are at a unique juncture in the history of weight loss. Up to now the condition or context in which people have been holding weight loss has been the Diet Mentality. All the established assumptions, points of view, and attitudes claim that the only way to lose weight is to diet. What makes that context so uncomfortable is the mounting evidence that it doesn't work. In addition, that context has created frustration, hopelessness, and anxiety. This book is about creating a new context or way of thinking about weight loss, a new approach and set of attitudes. It is a context that focuses on what *does* work rather than what doesn't work.

Here's an example of what I mean. Suppose the stereo system you really want costs $5,000. Which one of these approaches would work better:

● Worrying, fretting, and moaning about how you don't have $5,000?

- Concentrating on what you need to do to raise $5,000?

Of course, the second would work better, but in order for it to be successful, you would have to let go of the first entirely. You would have to let go of the old context in order to make room for the new. That's what you need to do with weight loss. You have to look at your own experience and get clear that diets are *never* going to work. Then and only then will you be able to move on and create an entirely new context for losing weight.

We're pioneers in this quest. Someday everyone is going to know or admit that diets don't work. There will be newspaper stories, magazine articles, and scientific papers about it. But that's not the case now. The world is operating from the context that the way to lose weight is to diet, just as the world used to operate from the context that man couldn't fly — until someone made the first breakthrough.

Making It Yours

This book has been carefully designed to let you produce specific and measurable results. It's intended to give you the experience of being a thin person that people get in my Diets Don't Work Seminars. It's your personal workbook, a private seminar that's yours and yours alone.

The exercises in each chapter are for your eyes only, unless you choose otherwise. They are a way for you to discover how the unwanted pounds got there in the first place, what has been in the way of taking them off, and what it will take for you to become a thin person once and for all.

Everyone who reads this book will discover different things about themselves. Your insights and realizations will be unique to you. Having these insights won't take off the weight, but it will allow you to see how it got there and why it stays.

In other words, reading this book may not prevent you from going on a binge, but it will help you find out what really sets you off and discover what to do about it. You'll be in a position to choose for yourself whether you want to live and eat like a fat person or like a thin person. You've never really been in a position to make that choice before because the Diet Mentality has obscured your thinking about being fat, and because you probably haven't had a direct experience of what it would be like to be thin. By working through the exercises, you will know by the time you get to the end of this book which choice you want to make.

Beginning to Be Your Own Best Friend

One of the most devastating things about the Diet Mentality is that it encourages you to hate yourself and your body and to treat yourself accordingly. The Diets Don't Work approach to the whole issue of weight is to be kind, positive, and gentle with yourself. Being overweight is not a crime. The person inside your body, the real you, is a capable, worthy individual and a beautiful being.

I invite you to put self-recrimination behind you and start now to be loving toward yourself. We're all indoctrinated with the idea that we have to use harsh discipline on ourselves to get results. In fact, just the opposite is true. It's time to start treating yourself like the wonderful being you are. It's time to start taking care of yourself as if you were a precious possession.

There are probably hundreds of ways you neglect yourself or treat yourself like a second-class person. In the next exercise you get to play the part of your best friend, someone who knows everything about you. You're going to make lists of all the things that, if someone did them for you, would make you feel cared about and appreciated. This is an extremely important exercise because we will use it in a later chapter. But the purpose of it right now is for you to get down in black and white all of the many ways in which you're not now treating yourself like a worthy person. Like not sewing on that missing button, or not applying for the job you really want, or not flossing your teeth everyday, or not treating yourself to a nice walk or a bubble bath. I've divided the list into five categories with space for five items under each category and included two exercises on incompletions.

EXERCISES (30 minutes)

1. "These are five personal things I would like to do for myself that would make me feel cared about:"

a.

b.

c.

d.

e.

2. "These are five things I would like to do for myself at work that would make me feel cared about:"

a.

b.

c.

d.

e.

3. "These are five things I would like to do around the house that would make me feel cared about:"

a.

b.

c.

d.

e.

4. "These are five things I would like to do in my relationships that would make me feel cared about:"

a.

b.

c.

d.

e.

5. "These are five things I would like to do about my body that would make me feel cared about:"

a.

b.

c.

d.

e.

6. "These are 100 incompletions I'm willing to complete or goals I'm willing to attain within the next three months (list anything that you began but did not finish, anything that you thought about doing but did not do, anything that's not complete for you — letters not written, buttons not sewed on, communications not delivered, etc.):"

1. _____

2. _____

3. _____

4. _____

5. _____

6. _____

7. _____

8. _____

9. _____

10. _____

11. _____

12. _____

13. _____

14. _____

15. _____

16. _____

17. _____

18. _____

19. _____

20. _____

21. _____

22. _____

23. _____

24. _____

25. _____

26. _____

27. _____

28. _____

29. _____

30. _____

31. _____

32. _____

33. _____

34. _____

35. _____

36. _____

37. _____

38. _____

39. _____

40. _____

41. _____

42. _____

43. _____

44. _____

45. _____

46. _____

47. _____

48. _____

49. _____

50. _____

51. _____

52. _____

53. _____

54. _____

55. _____

56. _____

57. _____

58. _____

59. _____

60. _____

61. _____

62. _____

63. _____

64. _____

65. _____

66. _____

67. _____

68. _____

69. _____

70. _____

71. _____

72. _____

73. _____

74. _____

75. _____

76. _____

77. _____

78. _____

79. _____

80. _____

81. _____

82. _____

83. _____

84. _____

85. _____

86. _____

87. _____

88. _____

89. _____

90. _____

91. _____

92. _____

93. _____

94. _____

95. _____

96. _____

97. _____

98. _____

99. _____

100. _____

7. "This is what I would give in order to have all those goals and dreams realized and all those incompletions complete..."

_____

_____

_____

_____

_____

The Fat and Thin Persons Inside You

Before we go on to Part II, "Dismantling the Diet Mentality," I want to prepare you for a battle that will be raging while you're reading this book. It is a battle between the fat person and thin person inside you. They represent two parts of yourself, and each has a voice.

The fat person is the one who says things like:

- "Go ahead, have that Danish pastry, you deserve it."
- "You were bad to eat that piece of pie."
- "You've already blown it, you might as well have the ice cream, too."
- "Let's wait till Monday before we start losing weight."
- "A neat guy like him wouldn't go out with a fat girl like you."

You haven't heard from the thin person much recently, but you'll begin to hear more from him as we go along.

Up to now the fat person has been winning — he's had a lot of experience, he's an expert in the Diet Mentality, and he knows exactly what to say to defeat you. As you've read along in this book, he's probably become more and more uncomfortable and restless. You're blowing his cover with every page you read. When you get him out into the light of day, you'll see that you're a lot bigger than he is and don't have to let him run your life.

He's not going to give up without a fight, though, so be prepared. We'll talk more about him as we go along. Remember that the more he screams and squirms, the closer you are to exposing him, to finding your own answers, to trusting yourself, to letting go of your negative self-image, to being free of the Diet Mentality.

The next part of the book will really bring out that negative voice. We'll take a look at what you're up against in losing weight and letting go of the Diet Mentality, you'll get a chance to be thin for a day, and by the end of Part II, you'll choose how you want to live the rest of your life.

Part II:
Dismantling The Diet Mentality

CHAPTER 4

Reasons Why You Overeat

Beating Yourself Up

This chapter is going to be a difficult one. Already 30 of every 100 people who started to read this book have quit. You're among the 70% who have stayed with it, who have had the courage and commitment to keep going. And it will take even more of your determination and commitment to get through this section of the process.

In this chapter we're going to look at some of the habits many of us have developed in relation to food, some of the ways we keep ourselves overweight. You're probably already familiar with some of those habits and with some of the reasons you eat that have nothing to do with giving your body the fuel it needs. As you read this chapter, you'll discover more.

But first I want to warn you that when people begin to examine what they've done in the past in relation to food, they have a tendency to become grim and use what they discover to punish themselves. It's important for you to remember that what you did then was probably appropriate or even necessary in its time and its place. In any case, you had to pass through that phase to get to where you are now. The past is past.

This book is designed to be a tool for learning how to be thin, not a whip for beating your fat body. It's like a microscope for observing yourself at close range. Let it be your servant, not your master. Let it support and encourage you forward.

As you read this chapter, you may see things about yourself that you don't particularly like. So what? You need that information in order to transform your relationship with your body. Before you can repair a watch, it helps to understand why it's broken. Before you can dismantle the Diet Mentality and take off your weight once and for all, it's important to understand how it got there and what makes it stay.

Everyone acts in ways that don't benefit them — yours just center around eating. And unlike some people, you have the courage to examine those habits and tell the truth about them. After recognizing what they are, you can work to change them.

Remember, the purpose of this book is not to make you a wise fat person or a grim fat person, but to end weight as a problem in your life forever. Being grim, on the other hand, is part of the Diet Mentality and only encourages the kind of negative attitude that gives rise to the cycles of weight loss and weight gain we've been talking about. People often think they have to be tough on themselves just to keep themselves in line. "Don't do that," "Don't eat that," "Don't you dare stop starving until you lose all your weight" are the hallmarks of the Diet Mentality. No matter how fast or far you go, it's never fast or far enough. Why devote your life to being miserable?

When you're gentle with yourself, the positive and creative aspects just bubble to the surface without any effort. It's like watering the flowers instead of the weeds. The attractive and thin person inside you will come forth when he or she knows that it's safe. A loving, accepting, nurturing environment will draw the thin person out much faster.

When you recognize yourself eating for one of the reasons we're going to mention, your tendency will be to think, "Oh no, I'm even worse than I thought." It's not necessary to do that. Just notice what you're doing and accept it for what it is. You simply chose some habits instead of others, and you can change them if you wish. There are worse things in life than eating for the wrong reasons. Reasons are neither positive nor negative in themselves, but only in so far as they support or hinder you in accomplishing your purpose — losing weight.

The Reasons for Eating

Sometimes I think overweight people are the most creative and imaginative people in the world. Every time we do a Diets Don't Work Seminar, someone comes up with a new answer to the question, "Why do you eat?" As you read through this list of reasons for eating, look honestly at your own life and check off the ones you've used in the past. If you come up with your own versions or examples, add them in the space provided. And don't worry about your score.

1. WARM FUZZIES. Sometimes there's nothing in the world as comforting as eating. It doesn't talk back to you. It doesn't withdraw its love. If something upsetting happens at the office, or you have a problem with your relationship, or even if you just feel depressed for no reason, eating will soften the pain, whether it's physical or emotional.

Yes ☐   No ☐

_____

_____

2. THE CONNOISSEUR. You love the taste of good food. That finely honed palate is always on the prowl. What if you miss eating something? It may be your last chance.

Yes ☐   No ☐

_____

_____

3. THE REWARD. You were so good today that you deserve to eat. You worked so hard, did such a good job at the office or with

the kids. God knows, it's time you did something for yourself. You have to reward yourself when you're good, don't you?

Maybe you've stuck to your diet all day long, and now it's 9:00 P.M. Surely you deserve a reward for that.

Or you've overcome some great trial, weathered some storm. You car battery was dead this morning and you had to have it recharged. That ought to be worth at least a package of Twinkies.

Or you spent your whole lunch hour talking to a friend who was depressed. Saints have to keep their strength up.

Or after all, you cooked it. Who has a better right to eat it?

Yes ☐   No ☐

---

4. THE STARVING CHILDREN IN CHINA. "Don't you dare leave a scrap of food on your plate when there are starving children in the world." You've heard it since you were two years old. (Mothers get reports each morning about where the children are starving that day.) It's a tape that plays in almost everyone's mind, consciously or unconsciously. You're not only selfish and spoiled, you threaten world peace and prosperity if you don't eat that last bite.

Another version of the Starving Children in China Game is the Clean Plate Club. In some families only the children who belong to the Clean Plate Club are allowed to get up from the table or have dessert. The rest have to sit there until they stuff every last piece of food on the plate into their overfed bodies.

When you can't leave anything on the plate now, you're probably not thinking about the starving children or the Clean Plate Club, but the rule is still in your mind. An empty plate is good, you believe, and it's bad to throw anything away.

Yes ☐   No ☐

Carol, who took the seminar in Oakland, told a wonderful story about the starving children habit. She was once at a breakfast meeting where someone had spread out dozens of assorted pastries and donuts on a huge platter. As she devoured one piece after another, the man sitting across from her, who was very thin, took a pecan roll, put in on his plate, and sat nibbling only the good parts off the top of it — the pecans, butter, and caramel. By the end of the meeting, much to her dismay, there was just a lump of dough left, with all the sweet, crunchy parts eaten off. When he got up to leave, she asked him if he wasn't going to eat the rest of it. Smiling sheepishly, he said, "I only like the top."

Was his leaving the roll on his plate any more of a waste than her stuffing one pastry after another into her overstuffed body? That moment was a revelation to Carol. She saw that putting something in your stomach doesn't keep it from being wasted, and that world hunger wasn't going to get any worse because that man hadn't eaten his whole pecan roll.

5. SLOGAN EATING. This game is closely akin to the Starving Children in China. Slogan eating comes from those bits of wisdom handed down to us at the dinner table like, "Take all you want, but eat all you take." The person who said it might not be standing over you any more, but the rule remains.

Yes ☐   No ☐

_____

_____

6. BARGAIN EATING. Someone else is paying for it, so why not? You might as well have the soup *and* the salad *and* the dessert. You don't get taken out to dinner every day, so you should get as much out of it as you can.

Or you've found this wonderful little market or restaurant where the prices are so low you can't resist. Who can pass up a bargain? Take the eclair. It's a steal. Take three! It's cheaper than *one* at the other place.

Or the place down the street has an "all you can eat" night every

Wednesday. You didn't want to go, but someone dragged you there. As long as you paid the whole price, you have to get more than your money's worth. Of course, to do that you'll have to have three or four helpings.

Or it's free. Free samples in the supermarket. Cookies and goodies at a party, or the free meal on the airplane. It doesn't matter. If it's free you've got to take it. Nothing's free anymore, so see how much you can eat.

Yes ☐   No ☐

_____

_____

7. GRAZING. Being from Texas, I like this one best. Sometimes when I had a project to do, I would lay out all my materials, and then I would decide that I wanted something to eat. I would go into the kitchen looking for *it*. I would see something that looked good and eat that. No, that wasn't it. Of course, I would keep going until I got to the other end of the kitchen, and by that time I'd have eaten so much that I would have to lie down. The project I was working on had to wait.

Yes ☐   No ☐

_____

_____

8. TV EATING. Sharon, who came to the seminar in Los Angeles, said that she never watched TV without eating, and never ate dinner without watching TV. She didn't even have a table in her kitchen or dining room, only a TV tray in front of her television. The two things, eating and TV, were completely locked together in her mind.

One week when her TV set was broken, she lost five pounds. "I just didn't have any desire for food unless I was watching TV," she said.

Sometimes TV-eating reaches such a fine art that there are different foods for different programs. Maybe some pasta with *As the World Turns* and chocolate cookies with the evening news.

Yes ☐   No ☐

_____

_____

9. SCARCITY EATING. Grab it now, because if you don't, someone else will. This is your last chance, you might not eat again for days. There will never be another strawberry shortcake like this one. You'd better take it while you can. A Scarcity Eater is like a lion feeding in the jungle.

Yes ☐   No ☐

_____

_____

10. THEY MADE ME DO IT. Your friend insisted you try the specialty at his favorite restaurant. Or you don't want to offend your hostess by not finishing dinner. It would be impolite to refuse a second helping, wouldn't it? You can't say no to people. You don't want to be rude. It's more important to be liked or get approval than to be thin.

You were going to go right home after the movie, but they insist you stop for pizza. And then they tell you they're too full to eat the last piece, so you have to finish it off.

Or you go home, and your mother has laid out enough food in the refrigerator to cater the Thirty Years War. She made it all for you, and you can't hurt her feelings by not eating it.

Yes ☐   No ☐

_____

_____

11. SOUVENIR EATING. You're away from home and you may never get back to that cute little restaurant in San Francisco. You eat as if you were collecting souvenirs, except when you get home you can't put them on the mantle — you've already put them on your hips.

Sometimes when I traveled to cities where the food was supposed to be particularly good, I would feel like a giant worm, eating my way from block to block.

Yes ☐   No ☐

_____

_____

12. HEALTH. You're bigger, so you need to eat more, right? If you don't, you'll get malnutrition. You'll get sick and have to go to the hospital.

"Feed a fever, starve a cold." Or is it the other way around? Best to be safe — feed them both.

If you stop eating, you'll start smoking again. Better to gain a few pounds than to die of lung cancer.

"I only ate junk food today, so I'd better eat something nutritious to balance it out."

Yes ☐   No ☐

_____

_____

13. PREVENTIVE EATING. If you don't eat now, you may get hungry later. And who knows if there will be anything to eat later? You'd better have another helping just in case.

I always used to eat just before getting on a plane because the airline food was supposed to be so bad. And those tiny portions! What if they served something up there that was terrible. I would be trapped 30,000 feet in the air with nothing to eat for hours. (As it turns out, I've never missed a meal on a plane.)

Yes ☐   No ☐

_____

_____

14. TRANSITION EATING. Eating divides up the day. It gives you permission to do what's next. Coffee and rolls means you're halfway to lunch. Lunch means you're halfway through the workday. Dinner means that work is over and you can relax and get on to your personal or social time. Eating can be a way of letting you know it's okay to go on the next part of your day.

Yes ☐   No ☐

_____

_____

15. PRE- AND POST-DIET EATING. Monday morning you're going to start on the new diet and make it work this time, even if you die in the process. It's Sunday night, a condemned person's last meal. What does it matter? You'll be taking it off anyway, or you'll be dead, so what difference does it make. Eat up all the temptations. Think of how good you're going to be tomorrow morning.

Or you've just come off a diet. You've spent a whole week picking at grapefruit and hard-boiled eggs, and now the thought of them makes you sick. Maybe you even lost a few pounds. You have a little leeway now, and besides, you'll never go back to eating the way you used to. Why not have just a *little* forbidden food to prove you can do it. You certainly deserve it.

Yes ☐   No ☐

_____

_____

16. PRE- AND POST-EXERCISE EATING. You need to keep your strength up if you're going to exercise. You'll probably faint right there in the gym if you don't have something to eat. Anyway, it will all come off when you work out.

After you exercise, you feel good. You burned off all those calories and you deserve something to eat.

Yes ☐   No ☐

_____

_____

17. CLOSET EATING. You eat for no better reason than that no one's watching. Most of the day there are people around. They're always watching you, probably adding up all the things you're eating and shaking their heads. Well, they aren't around now — hit the kitchen!

Or you go out with friends and have nothing but a salad. You're watching your weight after all, and they're watching *you*. They admire you and praise you for having such willpower. That's great, but when you get home you can't wait to get to the kitchen.

Yes ☐   No ☐

_____

_____

18. HOLY GRAIL EATING — THE QUEST FOR SATISFACTION. A woman named Karen, from Oakland, came up with this one. She said that she spent years looking for something in life that would really satisfy her. She didn't seem to be getting what she wanted from her job or her relationship, so she figured the best place to look for it was in the refrigerator. Every day she would open the refrigerator door and stare at the shelves, looking for something that would make her happy. She looked behind the mayonnaise, rustled around in the vegetable crisper, peered under the butter dish. All the time she would be popping things into her mouth.

When Karen finally found satisfaction, it wasn't in the kitchen or the refrigerator.

Yes ☐   No ☐

_____

_____

19. HUNGER PAINS. You have that funny feeling in your stomach and it starts to rumble. Your mother told you those were hunger pains, and you think, "Uh-oh. Better eat something quick, I'm having hunger pains!" That's not what's happening at all. We've never had hunger pains in our lives! It's not like having a headache in our stomach. We're just having hunger *feelings!*

Make a fist and look at its size. How much food would it take to fill it up? Well, that's how big your stomach is. But how much food do you eat? At least enough to stretch it out to a two-or three-fist size? When you stomach tries to shrink back down to normal, it makes those funny noises and has those feelings. It's healthy, and if you think about it, it feels pretty good. Hooray! Your stomach is shrinking! You should celebrate, not go out and see how much you can stuff into it.

Yes ☐   No ☐

_____

_____

In the Oakland seminar, a woman named Betty shared that when she was a child her mother told her that stomachs work by rubbing back and forth against the food. If there was no food in there, she was told, her stomach would then rub a hole in itself! As Betty grew older, she forgot this story. But every time she tried to cut down on her eating, she would become frightened that if she didn't eat, she would get sick. The feeling would become so strong that she would always eat, no matter how determined she was to lose weight.

20. I'M GROWN UP NOW, AND I'LL DO WHATEVER I WANT. When we were children, our parents had a lot of control over what we ate. Sometimes that made us mad, and we unconsciously adopted the point of view, "When I grow up and have my own money, I'm going to eat everything they wouldn't let me have." We spend the rest of our lives proving that no one can tell us what not to eat.

Yes ☐   No ☐

_____

_____

21. UNCONSCIOUS EATING. There are certain times, places, and situations in which you just eat as if part of you were an automatic eating machine. Each time you go to a movie, you head straight for the popcorn. The first bite is just wonderful. The second bite is pretty good, too. But after that you go unconscious, and next thing you know your hand is at the bottom of the box with a bunch of seeds. Most of us eat unconsciously 95% of the time.

Yes ☐   No ☐

_____

_____

22. BOREDOM EATING. You have time on your hands —
what are you supposed to do with it except eat? It takes time to eat,
after all. You have to think about what you want, go to the store
and buy it, then spend time fixing it, and finally you get to eat it.
Then you have to wash up and put everything away. There are
people who spend four to six hours a day repeating this ritual.
Eating is a way to fill their time.

It works in reverse, too. You don't have enough time, so you'd
better shove it all in while you can. Or you have so little time for
yourself that you should do whatever you want to do, and what's
more fun than eating?

Yes ☐   No ☐

_____

_____

23. WORRY EATING. Things aren't going well at all. You're
tense and anxious. You don't know exactly what it is, but something is wrong. What's the quickest, easiest way to stuff down those
feelings? Eat.

Or this is a time in your life that's upsetting. Maybe you're going
through a divorce, or the pressure is on at work, or you've had a
personal crisis. Instead of really experiencing the emotions you're
feeling, you push them down with food. The problem, of course, is
that they always come back, just as big or bigger than they were
before, because you haven't dealt with them.

Maybe you're in one particular situation that makes you nervous
— out to dinner with new people or with people you really don't
want to spend time with, at a party or at a big business meeting.
Any time you want to get rid of anxiety, all you have to do is stuff it
— literally. The only problem is that it always comes back.

Yes ☐   No ☐

_____

_____

24. CREATIVE EATING. You love to cook, and you're good at it. It's one of the ways you express yourself. You certainly can't be expected to give that up. And once you've cooked a glorious gourmet dinner, you can't be expected to toss it down the disposal, either. *Someone* has to eat it, right? It might as well be you.

Or you're into exploring new foods. It's part of your adventurous spirit, your zest for living, for discovering the finer things in life.

Yes ☐   No ☐

_____

_____

25. HOLIDAY EATING. It's Thanksgiving. You're expected to eat. Everyone overeats at Thanksgiving, even thin people. What would Thanksgiving be if you didn't eat yourself into a coma and have to lie down after dinner?

Christmas can be even worse because it lasts longer. With Thanksgiving it's over in a day. With Christmas it lasts for weeks. Holiday parties and family get-togethers. Eat, drink, and be merry. "Tis the season." Candies, cakes, drinks, buffets, family dinners. You don't want to spoil the holiday for everyone; you don't want to be a wet blanket. And anyway, that's what holidays are for — to celebrate. Who ever tried to lose weight during the holidays?

Yes ☐   No ☐

_____

_____

26. ENERGY EATING. You need energy if you're going to face this day, let alone get through it. And at night when you're tired, you have to fortify yourself with more food.

Or you're afraid you'll have too much energy if you don't eat.

Eating calms you, soothes you, keeps you on an even keel. If you don't eat, you'll get hyper and nervous.

Yes ☐   No ☐

---

27. RITUAL EATING. You can eat a certain thing at a certain time, or under certain circumstances, and you do it every day, no matter what. If the ritual is going across the street for a candy bar at 3:30, you'll do it even if it's hailing golf balls outside. If you don't eat when the ritual calls for it, you feel tremendously cheated.

I know a woman who always took her coffee break at 10:30. Every day she would walk down the street to a certain deli and buy a croissant, take it back to her desk, and eat it. Once the owner of the deli got sick and closed the store for a few days. She was beside herself. There were other places she could buy croissants, but they weren't the croissants that she wanted. She wanted the ritual, and nothing else would do.

Yes ☐   No ☐

---

28. PROCRASTINATION EATING. Did you ever get set to do a big project and find yourself drifting toward the kitchen? Some people procrastinate by staring into space. Others bite their fingernails. Others start cleaning the house. People with weight problems usually overeat.

Yes ☐   No ☐

---

29. GUILT EATING. It might have started with something as simple as getting up late or forgetting to make an important phone call. Or maybe you screamed at the kids, or made a mistake at work, or just didn't feel very good about yourself that day. How do you deal with the guilt? Eat. Now you can feel guilty about eating, too. You've blown it already, so why not sit down for a double helping at dinner.

Yes ☐   No ☐

_____

_____

30. LOVE FOOD. Whether you're falling in or out of it, love can lead to eating. It's easy to see why you'd eat if you were falling out of love, or if someone were falling out of love with you. It's the end of a relationship. You're unhappy, upset, anxious, confused, and hurt. You yearn for the comfort and temporary quiet that food can give you. It's not a happy time, and all you want is to go unconscious. Besides, now that it's over, who cares whether you look good or not?

It's not so obvious why people eat when they're falling *in* love. You would think they would be especially interested in *losing* weight. But falling in love is a happy and exciting time. It brings new feelings, including its own set of anxieties. Even though you've longed to have those feelings, they can be unfamiliar and disconcerting. One sure-fire way to tone them down is to eat.

Yes ☐   No ☐

_____

_____

There are more reasons people overeat. You probably know some that we haven't mentioned here. But this gives you a sampling so you can start to identify your own.

Now take ten more minutes and complete these exercises before you go on.

EXERCISES (10 minutes)

1. "These are the reasons I eat:" (To get answers, keep asking yourself, "Why do I eat?" or "Why do I overeat?")

a.

b.

c.

d.

e.

f.

g.

h.

2. "These are three reasons not mentioned in this chapter that I use for overeating:"

a.

b.

c.

3. "These are the payoffs or benefits I get from eating for these reasons:"
(Example: "I always overeat when I'm at my mother's house because I want to avoid a fight.")

a.

b.

c.

d.

e.

f.

g.

h.

4. "These are the specific circumstances in which I'm likely to overeat:"

a.

b.

c.

d.

e.

Behind the Reasons for Eating:
The Personal Laws

My purpose in having you look at the reasons you eat has been threefold. First, when you realize the extent to which you eat for head reasons rather than body reasons, you'll see that diets are never going to work because they leave those head reasons untouched — and hassle your body instead. Second, you have to look at those reasons in order to see the contrast between the Diet Mentality and the Naturally Thin Mentality and to see how out of touch with your body you probably are right now. And third, by examining those reasons in detail, you'll come to see that there are deeper reasons — what I call personal laws — that underly them.

In our seminars participants start getting in touch with those personal laws. Till then they're largely unconscious of them, and as long as that's the case, there's no way for them to gain mastery over them.

You may be wondering where those personal laws come from. They come from our experience, some event or events in our life that have caused us to make a decision about ourselves, about how to operate in life, about how to succeed or how to survive. Personal laws have their purpose, but when they become unconscious and start operating automatically, we're stuck with them long after they've stopped playing a useful function. Even worse, many of the most powerful personal laws were made when we were too young to have an accurate picture of who we are or of what the world is actually like, and so are often terribly misguided. In the case of eating, as long as we try to motivate ourselves with all kinds of very good reasons for losing weight but don't stop to really examine the underlying laws that keep us fat, we'll never become thin.

The big question is, how do you discover the reasons for your being overweight? First you need to look at the unwanted results you're producing. One of the rules of life I learned from Randy Revell of Context Trainings is that we always do what's most important to us. If you want to know what your priorities are, just look at what you do.

Then simply ask yourself what rules or personal laws you might have invented which would cause you to act the way you do. Just stay aware, keep asking yourself those questions, and eventually your personal laws will become clear to you.

Let me give you an example. Jane Springer, thirty-five years old and the mother of two, is trying to lose weight again, this time because of an upcoming wedding. This is what she has to say about being overweight.

> Oh I wish I were thin. I know I would feel so much better. Over the years I've tried every diet under the sun, but I just can't keep the weight off. It's such a battle. Overweight has been a problem since I was a young girl. Well, some of us are like that. My oldest daughter has the same problem. When she was young, I thought she was a cute, chubby, healthy, little girl. But now I see she's just like me, as I am like my mother. It runs in the family. My youngest child bothers me sometimes, he's so thin I'm afraid he'll be sickly and frail the rest of his life. I tell him how lucky he is that he doesn't have to worry about weight. I always reward him when he cleans his dinner plate; he gets a big bowl of ice cream. I should be so lucky...

Now what conscious and unconscious rules are motivating Jane?
- Thin people feel better than fat people.
- Dieting is very difficult.
- Weight loss can never be permanent.
- Being overweight has always been a problem, so it will continue to be a problem.
- Fat babies are healthy babies.
- The tendency to be overweight is inherited; there is really nothing one can do about it.
- Thin people are sickly, so who would want to be thin.
- Food is rewarding; clean your plate to get dessert.

Upon close examination it becomes clear that Jane has many conflicting rules and attitudes about weight that make weight loss difficult for her, attitudes that she's passing on to her children. For example, she truly believes that she has always had and will always have a weight problem. Her mother has one, her daughter has one — it runs in the family. Since she sincerely believes this to be true, her behavior — overeating — will produce results which support this belief. Jane is teaching her youngest child that food is a reward rather than nourishment. Most likely, he will continue to reward himself with food as he grows older — a snack after mowing the lawn, a piece of cake after giving his children a bath. If Jane becomes aware of her rules and attitudes, she can evaluate them and decide whether or not to continue using them.

You, too, have the same choices as Jane. You can continue to remain unaware of the basic rules and attitudes you have about your body, or you can make a conscious effort to discover what those rules and attitudes are. Once you know what motivates you to overeat then you can choose to do something fundamental about it. The exercises below are designed to stimulate your awareness — you may discover that there are a number of personal laws that dictate your eating habits. All of them may not become clear to you at once. In that case, these exercises will function like a time-release capsule, whose effects will be realized gradually, as you go along.

EXERCISES (20 minutes)

1. What were the circumstances in your life when you first began to gain weight? How old were you? What were your relationships like? What was your money situation? How successful were you in school or at work? Was there some trauma, crisis, or pressure in your life? Provide as much detail as possible.

2. Under what circumstances do you overeat today? Describe your cirumstances in deta   in exercise 1, above.

3. When you attempt to imagine yourself being thin, what objections come to mind? (For example: (a) "Good mothers aren't thin and sexy"; (b) "People might expect more from me"; (c) "My friends or family might not like it if I change"; (d) "I'll have to do all the things I said I would do if I ever got thin.")

4. Now look back over your answers to the foregoing questions and see if you can find the underlying laws that motivate you to overeat.

5. Look at your personal laws closely. Are they still useful or true? Do they reflect an accurate picture of your life as you now know it to be?

Why Thin People Eat

Have you ever asked thin people why they eat? When I have, they've eyed me suspiciously and said, "Is this some kind of trick question?" When I assured them that I really wanted to know, they've looked at me as if I were crazy and said, "I eat because I'm hungry."

You rarely get that answer from people with weight problems, and now you can begin to see why. After eating for all the other reasons, they never really know what it's like to be hungry.

When naturally thin people are hungry, they eat. They eat exactly what they want, but when their bodies have had enough, they stop. When they're not hungry, you can't force them to eat. We're so busy eating we very seldom get to the point of hunger. We eat because the food smells good or tastes good, because it might spoil if we don't eat it, or simply because it's there. We're like an eating machine that someone forgot to turn off.

Most of us use food to satisfy all kinds of appetites — emotional appetites, intellectual appetites, sexual appetites. We feel the craving and habitually assume it's for food. The problem is that those appetites never really get satisfied.

Barbara, from Houston, wrote me this letter after she finished the seminar:

> I was having dinner with a naturally thin friend last night, and we were discussing the weight problem of a mutual friend of ours. My thin friend was asking me questions about what it was like to go on a binge, and I was trying to explain to her what it was like.
>
> I realized in explaining it to her that on a binge food ceases to be food. When I went on a binge, I would attribute all kinds of abstract qualities to the food — safety, warmth, security, comfort, happiness. Looking back, I realize that I hardly tasted the food because it wasn't food anymore to me. It was the thing I wanted it to be at the time — like eating an abstraction. And since of course it really *was* only food, no amount of it would take the place of security, for example, or love, so I was never satisfied.
>
> The Diets Don't Work Seminar completely transformed all of that for me. Food doesn't have those

abstract qualities anymore, it's just food now. Since the
workshop I still eat to feel better and have been shocked
to discover that I don't feel better. I just feel fuller!

Suppose you had a naturally thin friend who was heart broken
because she'd just broken up with her boyfriend. As she sat there
crying, you reached out in compassion and offered her a donut.
What do you suppose she would do?

She would probably look at you and then look at the donut,
trying to figure out what you were doing. Perhaps she would ask
you if there was some kind of drug in the donut. But no, you assure
her it's just a regular donut. At this point she would probably ask in
desperation, "But what am I supposed to do with it?"

You see, to her food is something you put into your body when
you're hungry, the fuel you use to keep your body going. She
doesn't understand about food and problem solving. She doesn't
confuse physical and emotional appetites.

At one of the followup sessions of the Diets Don't Work Seminar, a woman named Pam, from San Francisco, told this story:

Last week I found myself walking around the kitchen
with a book in my hands. I realized halfway across the
kitchen that what I wanted most was to curl up and read.
What was I doing in the kitchen? I don't even have a
place to sit down in my kitchen. So I got a glass of water
and then went and curled up with the book. I began to
realize that hunger is a broad category for me, that it
covers the need for rest, the need for entertainment, the
need for affection, the need for many things that have
nothing to do with food.

Let's examine some of those appetites.

EXERCISES (3 minutes)

1. "These are the different emotional appetites I try to satisfy with
food:"

a.

b.

c.

d.

e.

2. "These are the specific foods I use to try to satisfy those appetites:"

a.

b.

c.

d.

e.

CHAPTER 5

Why You Can't Get There From Here

In the last chapter we described some of the reasons people eat. In this chapter we're going to look at some of the reasons you may have had for losing weight in the past and see what they have to do with your staying overweight.

Then we'll examine some of the reasons you may have had for *not* losing weight in the past and see what they all have in common. After we do that, it should become very clear why up to now the weight-loss game has seemed like a puzzle without a solution.

The Reasons for Losing Weight

As you read this section, see if you've used any of these reasons. If you have, check them off as you go along. If you have anything to add, write it in under your yes or no answer. Be as specific as possible. If you discover what you've been doing in the past that hasn't worked, it will be easier to change it and do the things that do work.

1. TO LOOK BETTER. No denying it — you would be more

attractive without the weight. You're not so bad now, but without those pounds you would look wonderful.

Yes ☐   No ☐

_____

_____

2. FOR THE BIG EVENT. It could be a party, a vacation, a class reunion, a date, going home to visit your family, any occasion where you want to look your best. You plan to lose the weight right before you go so you won't have a chance to gain it back.

Yes ☐   No ☐

_____

_____

3. RELATIONSHIPS. You want to get back down to your "hunting weight." It's time to get out there and meet new people or rekindle your present relationship.

Yes ☐   No ☐

_____

_____

4. HABIT. Life is an endless diet. You wouldn't know what to do with yourself if you gave up the quest for thinness. You've always wanted to lose weight, and if you stopped trying, just think

how bad it would get. You don't even think about going on a diet
anymore — you just do it as a matter of course.

Yes ☐   No ☐

_____

_____

5. TO GET ATTENTION. When you go out to lunch with
friends, you can sigh and look saintly, glance up to the heavens,
and tell them you're trying to lose weight. They'll feel sorry for
you and ask you all about it. "What kind of a diet is it? How does it
work?" If you didn't have this problem, you might have to spend
the whole lunch talking about them.

Yes ☐   No ☐

_____

_____

6. TO GET A JOB OR A PROMOTION. You're going to
breeze into that office looking like a stick, and they won't be able to
resist.

Yes ☐   No ☐

_____

_____

7. CLOTHING. The button that popped last week was the first
clue. Time to knock off a few pounds or you won't be able to wear

your clothes. You'll have to buy a whole new wardrobe.

Or maybe you want to buy a new wardrobe, but many sizes smaller.

Yes ☐   No ☐

_____

_____

8. IT'S SUMMER. Uh-oh. Sunbathing. Bikinis. The beach with all those semi-naked bodies — including yours. Big sweaters and baggy slacks don't make it in the summer.

Yes ☐   No ☐

_____

_____

9. LIFE IS GOING TO BE WONDERFUL. You'll finally cross the river into Happyland, where all the thin people live. Everything over there is just great. All will be perfect.

Yes ☐   No ☐

_____

_____

10. TO GAIN SELF-CONFIDENCE. Boy, when you get thin, the world had better watch out. You'll be a dynamo. Nothing will

be able to stop you. Then you'll be able to go anywhere and get exactly what you want.

Yes ☐   No ☐

_____

_____

11. TO PROVE YOU CAN. Whether you're proving it to yourself or to other people, someone is going to know that you can do it. Everyone is beginning to think you can't, after all these years. It was starting to be too much for your pride. You'll show them.

Yes ☐   No ☐

_____

_____

12. TO WIN A BET. A way to get thin and a little richer at the same time!

Yes ☐   No ☐

_____

_____

13. TO BE HEALTHIER. No more worrying about all those diseases and conditions you thought the weight might be fostering. You'll be the perfect specimen of health, and just wait until you get back on the tennis court. You'll live to be a hundred.

Yes ☐   No ☐

_____

_____

14. TO STOP THE NAGGING. Boy, are you tired of that! It would be worth it just to shut people up.

Yes ☐   No ☐

_____

_____

15. TO START EATING AGAIN. You fantasize about how you'll look when you've lost all that weight. And where do you picture yourself? In an ice cream parlor, sitting down to the biggest banana split ever concocted. When you're thin, you'll be able to eat anything you want without feeling guilty. Pizzas every night with pitchers of beer. Aahh!

Yes ☐   No ☐

_____

_____

16. TO END THE MISERY. Life isn't worth living if you have to live like this. Every day you feel worse about yourself. You hate the way you look, and you're such a creep you don't do anything about it. You'll do anything to stop feeling so miserable.

Yes ☐   No ☐

_____

_____

17. THE DOCTOR. Either he already told you that you had to lose weight, or you have an appointment scheduled. You know he's going to make you get' on the scale, and you can just see his eyebrows rising.

Yes ☐   No ☐

_____

_____

18. A SPECIAL PERSON. This is your big chance. If you blow it with this person, there may never be another. Besides, you want to please him or her. If ever there were a time to do it, it's now.

Yes ☐   No ☐

_____

_____

19. TO BE BETTER AT SPORTS. You used to be a terrific tennis player. You still have a great backhand, but somehow you can never get to the ball in time. Having twenty or thirty fewer pounds to lug around might make it easier.

Yes ☐   No ☐

_____

_____

20. TO LOOK YOUNGER. When people see a picture of your face, they think you're one age, but when they see a picture of your

whole body, they guess fifteen years older. The fat is making you look old before your time.

Yes ☐   No ☐

_____

_____

EXERCISES (3 minutes)

1. Make a list of other reasons we haven't mentioned here that have really motivated you to lose weight in the past.

a.

b.

c.

d.

e.

2. "These are the obstacles I've come up against in the past when I've tried to have the body I wanted:"

a.

b.

c.

d.

e.

The reasons for losing weight vary greatly. Some are internal, and some are external. Some are selfish, and others are not. Some seem real, others silly.

And they all have only one thing in common: they don't work. If they did, you would have already lost all your excess weight and kept it off. They're good reasons, but they're not good enough.

The Reasons For Not Losing Weight

Now let's look at why you may *not* have wanted to lose weight in the past.

1. YOU'RE GOOD, ABLE, AND ATTRACTIVE ENOUGH ALREADY. You don't have to lose weight to prove it. If they don't like you the way you are, who needs them?

Yes ☐   No ☐

_____

_____

2. TO PROVE SOMEONE WRONG. If they've shaken their heads and told you, as I used to tell people, that all you have to do is follow the diet and you'll be thin, then you can prove to them that it's not as easy as they think. You have a far more serious problem here than they'd imagined, and you're going to let them know it.

Yes ☐   No ☐

_____

_____

3. PEOPLE WOULD LEAVE YOU. They would be so envious of your beautiful new body that they wouldn't want to have anything to do with you. You would be all alone in the world.

Yes ☐   No ☐

_____

_____

4. THE WEIGHT WOULD JUST COME BACK. Once you lose it, there's no way to keep it off, so why make yourself miserable trying? It's hopeless.

Yes ☐   No ☐

_____

_____

5. MONEY. You would have to buy a whole new wardrobe. Everything you own would be hanging around your knees. At today's prices it'll cost a small fortune, and you don't have the money to do that right now. Better wait until you get a raise.

Yes ☐   No ☐

_____

_____

6. WHAT WOULD YOU DO WITH YOURSELF? What would you talk about, worry about, read about, plot about? How would you occupy your time if weight and food were no longer the big issues of your life?

Yes ☐   No ☐

_____

_____

7. IF YOU'RE MARRIED, IT'S SAFER TO BE FAT. What if the whole town were after your slender body? You don't want to ruin your present relationship, do you?

Yes ☐   No ☐

_____

_____

8. THERE WOULD BE NO MORE EXCUSES. If you lost the weight, you would have to confront relationships, success, and all those things on your "after I lose weight" list. Now you can blame the fat for not having those things. Listen, you can blame

almost anything on fat. It covers a multitude of sins, and who wants to blow a convenient excuse?

Yes ☐   No ☐

_____

_____

9. YOU LIKE YOURSELF JUST THE WAY YOU ARE. So why change?

Yes ☐   No ☐

_____

_____

10. IT WON'T MAKE ANY DIFFERENCE ANYWAY. You're wise to the ways of the world. You know being thin doesn't mean being happy. What's the point of losing weight and putting yourself through that agony if everything is going to be the same?

Yes ☐   No ☐

_____

_____

11. DISCIPLINE IS HARD. What a drag! There are enough problems in life without discipline. Besides, you don't think discipline is exactly your strong point. What if you try and fail again?

Yes ☐   No ☐

_____

_____

12. FEELING ROOTED AND STRONG. If the weight were gone, they would get you in a dark alley, for sure. People know you're around now, and they don't mess with you. You occupy space in the world. You're substantial, here to stay.

Yes ☐   No ☐

_____

_____

13. HEALTH. Losing and gaining weight again and again can actually cause health problems. Look at Mario Lanza, the famous opera singer — they say that's what killed him. Better to stay as you are than to get back on the roller coaster.

Yes ☐   No ☐

_____

_____

14. YOU CAN SAY PEOPLE REJECT YOU FOR YOUR FAT, AND NOT FOR WHO YOU ARE. It's another great excuse. If someone doesn't like you or leaves you, you can say they're leaving your fat body and not the real you.

Yes ☐   No ☐

_____

_____

15. THERE MIGHT BE AN EVEN BIGGER PROBLEM WAITING. The fat problem is familiar, we all know how to handle

it — we complain about it! If it were to disappear, there might be an even bigger problem waiting in the wings. Keep the fat around, and you get to keep the other problem waiting forever.

Yes ☐   No ☐

_____

_____

16. TO PUNISH SOMEONE. If someone doesn't like that you're fat, they've handed you the perfect weapon. Any time they step out of line, you can just head for the refrigerator.

Yes ☐   No ☐

_____

_____

EXERCISES (15 minutes)

1. Make a list of any other good reasons that have prevented you from losing weight in the past and that we haven't listed.

a.

b.

c.

d.

e.

f.

2. "In reading over the reasons given in this book and my own list, I see that these are the primary reasons I've had for not losing weight in the past:"

a.

b.

c.

d.

e.

f.

3. "These are all the fears I can think of that may be stopping me from losing weight:"

a.

b.

c.

d.

e.

f.

4. "This is what I think it would take for me to break through those reasons and fears:"

a.

b.

c.

d.

e.

5. "This is the first step I would have to take:"

6. "This is the next step:"

What do all these reasons for *not* losing weight have in common? *They work!* Now we've taken a major step forward — we're starting to recognize what works and what doesn't.

A Puzzle Without a Solution?

What do we have so far? In brief summary, this is what we've discovered:

- Diets don't work as a way to lose weight. They're great for gaining weight, though.
- Nobody seems to know what does work for losing weight.
- The reasons we eat are infinite in number (and very few of them have anything to do with hunger).
- All of them cause you to gain weight, and some of the payoffs are terrific.

- None of your reasons for losing weight have worked for you.
- All of your reasons for not losing weight have worked very well indeed.

Looks pretty hopeless, doesn't it? There seems to be no solution to the problem, in fact you could easily tie yourself into knots trying to lose weight. It's a game that can't be won. There's no way for you to get there from here.

Now, if you can't get there from here, it means you've been heading in the wrong direction. We've already seen that that's true. Everyone begins with the Diet Mentality, and with that as your starting point, you can never become thin.

If you're going to get anywhere at all, you're going to have to make a complete and dramatic shift in context, in your fundamental attitudes and points of view about your weight. In order to make that shift, you'll have to give up every notion you've ever had about losing weight, give up your ideas about what works and what doesn't work, and forget everything that's happened in the past.

In the next chapter we'll take a look at how a naturally thin person relates to food, and you'll get to experience what it's like to be thin for a day. This will give you a new outlook, a new perspective, on the whole issue of weight as a problem.

CHAPTER 6

How Thin People Think and Eat

The Secret

Are you ready for the big secret? Are you ready to find out how thin people can eat whatever and whenever they want without gaining weight? It's going to sound deceptively simple, but don't be fooled. It's the simplest and yet the most difficult thing in the world.

What makes it difficult is that it involves some basic, fundamental shifts in how you approach food, eating, yourself, and your life. As you read, imagine yourself behind that thin person's eyes, and notice how you feel.

In studying thin people, I learned that they do four fundamental things that fat people don't.

1. They hardly ever eat unless they are hungry.
2. They eat exactly what they want to eat.
3. They don't eat unconsciously; they stay conscious of what they're eating and the effect it's having on their body.
4. They stop eating when their body has had enough.

It's as simple as that. We couldn't believe it at first and tried to make it more complicated. It had to be the kind of food they ate or the time they ate it or their metabolism. But we found that some thin people eat junk food, and some eat health food. Some eat an early dinner, and some eat late at night. Some eat quickly, others eat slowly. The only things they all have in common are that they eat when they're hungry, they eat exactly what they want, they're aware of every bite they take and the effect it's having on their body, and they stop when their body has had enough.

If you stop to think about it, that's how children and animals eat. It's the natural approach to eating. Let's take those four characteristics one at a time.

1. THIN PEOPLE EAT BECAUSE THEY'RE HUNGRY. It doesn't occur to naturally thin people to combine donuts and sadness, as fat people often do. Their days don't revolve around food. Sometimes they say, "Oh, I forgot to eat today." The only time *we* forget to eat is when we're asleep or unconscious, but if thin people aren't hungry, they don't think about food. It isn't an issue in their lives, since they give themselves permission to eat exactly what they want.

It wouldn't occur to them to eat for any of the reasons we do — they eat because they're hungry, and what they eat tastes good to them. They don't waste food by eating more than their body needs. Food isn't a pastime or a hobby with them.

2. THIN PEOPLE EAT EXACTLY WHAT THEY WANT TO EAT. Thin people do a funny thing — before they sit down to a meal, they usually take the time to ask themselves what they want to eat. Grazing (see Chapter 4) is a foreign concept to them. They look to see what they want *before* they start eating.

They don't ask themselves what they *should* eat; they ask themselves what they want to eat. They seem to have some sort of inner barometer that tells them not only what would taste good at that particular moment, but also what their body wants and needs.

They know that if they want french fries, hard-boiled eggs aren't going to satisfy them. If they really want a baked potato, cottage cheese isn't going to do it. *If you want Rocky Road ice cream, a thousand carrot sticks aren't going to satisfy you!*

Normally, thin people are finicky eaters — they don't eat what they don't want. They don't eat just to be eating; they eat because a particular food rings a loud bell for them.

If they're out to lunch and nothing on the menu sounds tantalizing, either they'll leave and go elsewhere, or they'll order a token serving because they think it would be bad manners to sit in a restaurant without ordering something.

They do strange things, like not finishing everything on their plate. If a plate containing meat, vegetables, and potatoes is set in front of them, they'll only eat what they like. They may eat just the meat and the spinach, for example, and leave behind a mound of mashed potatoes. Or they may not touch the meat and eat a big dessert instead. Sometimes, if they have the option, they may not eat at all. They'll do something else instead. They know there will always be another meal.

And there's one thing naturally thin people never do — they never go on a diet.

3. THIN PEOPLE EAT CONSCIOUSLY. They stay conscious of what they're eating and the effect it's having on their body. They would never find themselves with their hand at the bottom of the box, wondering who ate all the popcorn. Since they pay attention to what they're eating, they're satisfied with less and enjoy their food more.

A man named Steve, from Houston, once told me that whenever he tried to get his son to finish the food on his plate, the boy would say, "I'm tired of eating!" We never get tired of eating because we're so used to doing it unconsciously. It's like driving a stick shift. When we are first learning and need to pay attention to what we're doing, it requires a great deal of effort. But after a while it becomes second nature, and we do it without thinking.

Because thin people are awake and conscious when they're eating, they know when their body has had enough. Most fat people have no idea how full they are before, while, or after they eat. Thin people keep tuned to their bodies, and they know when they're full.

Naturally thin people are ignorant about food. They don't know anything about diets, and the process of counting calories baffles them. They only know four things: when they're hungry, what they want to eat, what each bite of food they put in their mouth is doing there, and when they've had enough. When you think about it, that's all you really need to know in order to transform your Diet Mentality into a Naturally Thin Mentality.

EXERCISES (6 minutes)

1. "These are the fears I have about eating only when I'm hungry:"

a.

b.

c.

d.

e.

2. "These are the fears I have about eating exactly what I want:"

a.

b.

c.

d.

e.

3. "These are the things that might prevent me from stopping eating when my body has had enough:"

a.

b.

c.

d.

e.

4. "These are my fears about what would happen if I stayed conscious with every bite I ate:"

a.

b.

c.

d.

e.

5. "This is the amount of value in dollars that I have created for myself by reading this book so far:" $_____ .

4.   THIN PEOPLE STOP EATING WHEN THEIR BODY HAS HAD ENOUGH. Did you ever have someone try to press more food on you, even when you told them, "I'm on a diet?" Thin people have two words that stop people dead. They say, "I'm full," and if pressed, they just keep repeating it.

I've seen thin people stop eating right in the middle of an expensive meal and feel no guilt whatsoever. I've seen them wrap up and save one bite of food, or take all but two sips of a soft drink and put it back in the refrigerator. When you ask them why they don't finish it, they say, "I'm full. I'll eat it later." Doggie bags were invented for thin people. Fat people eat everything that lands on the table.

Naturally thin people don't care whether or not they're in the Clean Plate Club. They will occasionally overeat, but they don't give it a second thought. They treat food as if it were their servant, not their master. They don't pay a lot of attention to it. They will insult it, ignore it, leave it sitting on a plate, and even throw it away.

Portrait of a Thin Eater

Who are these people who are so ignorant they don't know the number of calories in a chocolate chip cookie, who don't even know what they do to stay thin? Why are naturally thin people like that, and how did they get that way?

The answer is that they didn't do anything and they don't know anything — that's just the point. Being thin is a natural state. We are the ones who have done something, who had added something to nature. We're the ones who have created the myths and the patterns and the rules that make and keep us fat. Take those away, and what you have is a natural state — *thin*. The Thins are like animals in the wild, following their body's instincts from moment to moment. We are the ones who have done something out of the ordinary.

It's not that thin people don't enjoy food — they do. They probably enjoy it more than we do, because they actually taste it. I used to buy ice cream cones, and the first bite would taste just great. After the second or third bite, I couldn't taste the flavor anymore — all I tasted was cold. If a thin person stopped enjoying the ice cream, he would probably toss the rest of it away.

It doesn't occur to thin people to use food as a reward. They reward themselves with other things. You see, in order to be effective, a reward has to be just a little bit naughty. Thin people sometimes think it's naughty to take the morning off to play tennis or to spend more money than they should on a new pair of slacks, but since they don't find food even the slightest bit wicked, it's of no use to them as a reward. They can't use it as a weapon against themselves or others. To them eating is like breathing — neither good nor bad.

They don't graze because they always have something particular in mind when they eat. They go after a specific food, rather than food in the abstract. They don't indulge in scarcity eating because it never occurs to them that someone might take their food away. And if they took it away, so what? There's always more. Thin people believe that food is all around them, there for the taking whenever they want it, so they never feel deprived. They have permission from themselves to eat whatever they want, whenever they want it, so what's the hurry?

Thin people also have this funny point of view that what their body tells them to eat is exactly what they need to stay healthy.

Usually, they don't worry too much about nutritional value. They know it will all work out in the end. If all they want to eat on a certain day is three chocolate bars, that's what they have. They may not get the chocolate craving again for a month. Because they give themselves permission to eat the chocolate when they want it, the craving goes away. The next day, they may only want vegetables or meat or bread. They trust their body's instincts, even when those instincts seem crazy.

I know one naturally thin person who is normally a vegetarian, but about every three months she gets an insatiable craving for two Big Macs, a large order of fries, and a chocolate shake. Nothing tastes good until she has that. When she feels the urge coming on, she heads straight for McDonalds. She just shrugs her shoulders and says, "My body wants it."

If a thin person can't remember whether it's "starve a fever, feed a cold" or the other way around, she won't starve them both. She'll just ask herself, "Does my body feel like eating or not?"

Some thin people actually enjoy the feeling of being hungry. Nadine, from Aspen, told me, "I feel so alive, as if I could beat Chris Evert at tennis. I have so much energy and think so clearly."

Thin people never indulge in closet eating. They don't have anything to hide. In fact, they often do the opposite. They're actually more likely to eat when someone's watching and may even eat more in a restaurant or when they're out to dinner with other people than they do when they're at home alone. It's a mystery to people who are overweight how a thin person can sit down and devour an enormous meal. The answer is that tomorrow *they might not eat anything.*

When thin people are anxious, they're more likely to undereat than to overeat. They don't know about the trick of burying their emotions under food. They may do something else — pace back and forth, sleep more than they normally do, go to a movie, or stare off into space — but when they're upset, food is often the farthest thing from their mind. They're too preoccupied to eat. Whatever is upsetting them has priority, and they can't even think about food.

It's not that thin people don't have problems, it's just that they don't make the connection between problems and food. Food is either neutral to them, fuel they use to keep their body functioning, or it's their friend. Thin people don't feel deprived, because they're not only eating what they want, they're doing the things that make them happy.

Are you beginning to get behind a thin person's eyes and see his approach to eating and food? That's what's important. This process is not just about doing the four things thin people do that fat people don't. It's about seeing where those four things come from and duplicating the thin person's mentality. If you don't change your basic attitude, you won't be any better off than if you'd gone on a diet. You'll just be left with another list of things you have to do to fix the situation you've gotten yourself into.

The trick is to start thinking like a thin person, feeling like a thin person, and behaving like a thin person. Be a thin person right now, and do it naturally. You'll have to change the self-image you've had for a long time, and you may have to pretend at first, until the new "rules" start to take hold.

What you will be doing is creating an environment in which the naturally thin person inside you feels comfortable and starts to emerge. The more you can allow that to happen, the more this new mentality will truly be yours. You will be a thin person inside, and it's only a matter of time before your body reflects who you really are.

Sharon, who took the seminar in Los Angeles, wrote:

> The first few days I couldn't believe how scarey it was to live like a thin person. It was almost as if there was too much freedom. Then I started exploring some of the things I could do with that freedom — like actually enjoying going out to dinner and getting off my own back about what I was going to eat — and it was great! I'm taking it step by step now and discovering a whole new world I never knew existed.

Just as you can't try to put a thin body underneath a fat head, you can't keep a fat body underneath a thin head for long. The more able you are to think like a thin person, the more effortless it will be for your body to follow suit. You won't have to think about it or worry about it. All you'll have to do is enjoy being thin. You didn't have to diet to gain the weight. It's only fair that you shouldn't have to diet to lose it.

EXERCISES (5 minutes)

1. Lean back, close your eyes, and visualize yourself as a thin person. Take yourself through a typical day, noticing what you would do, how you would interact with people, and how you would

eat. Create it exactly the way you want it to be. Take at least three minutes to do the exercise.

2. "These are the things that would be different about my life and about my relationship with myself and other people if I allowed myself to live as a thin person:"

a.

b.

c.

d.

e.

3. "On a scale of 1 to 10, this is how I would rate my certainty that I will actually become that thin person: _____ ." (10 = absolutely certain; 5 = maybe; 1 = never.) Todays date: _____ .

Thin for a Day: A Taste of the Thin Life

The best way for you to learn how thin people operate is to experience a day of approaching food the way they do. In my seminar I actually serve the participants lunch and dinner, during which we go through certain exercises to emphasize the Thin Mentality about food. I would like you to choose a day of relative freedom, say a Saturday or a Sunday, and recreate the experience for yourself, eating meals the way a thin person would and spending the day in the Thin Mentality.

In order to actually experience the Thin Mentality, there are several things you will need to know. I will explore each of these matters in more detail in Part III of this book, but for the purposes of this exercise, a brief introduction to *thin eating* is all that is necessary.

1. RATING YOUR HUNGER. Since you probably don't have a very clear idea of what it feels like to be hungry, I've devised a hunger scale, with 1 at the bottom and 10 at the top. One is when you're so hungry you feel faint. Ten is when you're so stuffed you can hardly move. Exactly in the middle, at 5 on the scale, is the point at which your body has had enough to eat. Everything up to 4.99 is "hungry"; everything from 5.01 on up is "overeating," "too much."

2. DISCONNECTING THE EATING MACHINE. In order to follow the third principle of thin eating, that is, eating consciously, you have to know how to get yourself off automatic. I call it disconnecting the eating machine. The object is to keep your attention on the food that's already in your mouth, so you actually taste it. To achieve this I have the people in my seminars put their fork down before they start to chew. Then I have them completely chew the bite that's in their mouth and swallow it before picking up their fork again.

3. SIZING UP YOUR STOMACH. Before we begin the meal in the seminar, I have everyone take their right hand and make a fist with it. This is the approximate size of your stomach when it has shrunk down to normal size. All those rumblings and grumblings

we experience are largely the result of the stomach trying to return to this size. If you're completely empty, the volume of food you need to eat to satisfy your body's hunger would fill a container the size of your fist.

4. RATING FOOD. Another thing you'll need to know before spending the day as a thin eater is how to rate food. Naturally thin people generally only eat foods they really love. So I've developed a food-rating scale, again from 1 to 10, with the numbers on the bottom of the scale representing your least-favorite foods and those at the top of the scale your favorite foods of all time. Foods at the level of 1 or 2 probably have no business being in your mouth. Naturally thin people generally only eat foods that are 9s or 10s for them. This is entirely a matter of taste; everybody has different preferences.

10	Wonderful, 'Orgasmic'
9	
8	Pretty Good
7	
6	OK, but Not Quality
5	
4	Not Good
3	
2	UGH!
1	

5. GETTING IN THE MOOD. Since you don't have the advantage of being in a seminar room where every aspect of your meals is controlled, you will need to know some things about how to approach eating on your thin day. The first thing is to treat yourself like a special person for that whole day. When you sit down to eat your meals, pretend you're an honored guest and someone has gone to a great deal of trouble to prepare a delicious meal for you. In the seminar we dim the lights in the room and play soft, relaxing music.

These will probably be the most special meals you will ever eat. You may want to eat them alone, so you can concentrate on the process of eating them like a thin person. If you do eat with someone, make sure that person is participating with you, supporting you in doing the exercise.

6. DOING WHAT THIN PEOPLE DO WHEN THEY'RE NOT EATING. Look back at your list of incompletions and goals that you compiled in Chapter 3. Pick out twenty incompletions you would like to complete during your first thin day. You probably won't come close to completing all twenty. That's not the object of this exercise, so don't get on your own case if you only get half of them done. The point is to do the things a thin person might do rather than think about food or weight.

7. WHAT TO EAT? Go ahead and have what you consider a light breakfast on your thin day. Then for lunch and dinner either prepare the same menu I offer in the seminars (listed below), or make up your own, but don't eat or drink anything except water between meals.

In order to make the exercise a success, choose a large variety of foods, including items you would ranks as 9s or 10s, as well as items that might be 3s or 4s. I recommend that you use as much fresh food as possible, and keep the quantities approximately the same as in the suggested menu. The following is the menu I serve:

Lunch:
  Fresh fruit (six or seven varieties, depending on what's in season: apples, oranges, bananas, fresh strawberries, pineapple, papaya, watermelon, grapes, etc.).
  Fresh (not dietetic) cottage cheese (2/3 cup).

Dinner:
  Half an avocado sandwich (brown bread, mayonnaise, slice of cheese, ½ avocado, alfalfa sprouts)
    Tomato (2 slices)
    Lettuce (2 leaves)
    Dill Pickle (1 slice)
    Dry-roasted Peanuts (20)
    Cheddar Cheese (1 cube)
    Swiss Cheese (1 cube)
    Brownie (1)

Before lunch, read through the following procedure, and follow it step by step.

PROCEDURE:

1. At about 1:00 p.m. check your level of hunger, and write

down what you think it is:_____ . (To do this, feel your stomach and guess what level between 1 [starving] and 5 [your body isn't hungry] you're experiencing. At this time you will eat lunch regardless of your hunger level.)

2. Set the table and prepare your plate as if you were serving a very special person. Use your favorite china and silverware. Set out flowers and candles, if you like. Turn on soft music.

3. Sit down and get ready. Before you start, pick up your plate and look at each item as if you'd never seen it before. Pretend it's from another world, even though it might look like something you've eaten before. Now smell each item. Can you determine from the smell what it might taste like? Remember, everything on your plate was a living entity just a short while ago and gave up its life for your pleasure. Treat each morsel of food with respect.

4. Now pick up one of the items with your fork, raise it slowly to your nose, and smell it. Closely examine what it looks like. Now put the food into your mouth, but before you begin to chew, *disconnect the eating machine.* Put your fork down on the plate.

5. Before starting to chew, suck on this morsel of food for a moment. Move it around in your mouth. See if you don't notice different flavors when it's in different parts of your mouth.

6. Now bite down on the food. Notice the sound it makes. Chew it very slowly, and continue to suck on it after every few chews.

7. After you've swallowed it, notice the aftertaste in your mouth. Do you like the taste? How would you rate it on a scale of 1 to 10?

8. Now go around the plate, eating one bite of each food on the plate in the same manner as you did the first. Notice how much you like each item.

9. After you've tasted every item on the plate once, put your fork down, pause a moment, and look at the food again. Which of the foods were 10s for you, and which were 1s?

10. Check your level of hunger before you continue.

11. Now eat the meal to satisfy your remaining hunger. Eat slowly, smell each bite before putting it into your mouth, and put your fork down before beginning to chew. Eat only the foods on the plate that are 8s, 9s, or 10s for you.

12. Stop eating for a few minutes, and do something your mother told you never to do — play with your food. Rearrange it on the plate. Make a design out of it.

13. As you complete the meal, keep checking your level of

hunger. If you're not sure whether your body has had enough food, give yourself permission to eat three more bites, then stop for a moment, check your hunger level again, and continue.

14. When you've reached a 5 on the hunger scale, put your fork down and stop eating. Pause a moment to notice what your body is experiencing; now look at what your mind is experiencing. Is the fat person talking to you? What is he saying?

15. Now comes the really hard part. Pick up your plate, carry it to the garbage can, and discard the remaining food. Say goodbye to the food and thank it for giving itself to you. Notice how you feel about throwing food away instead of stuffing it into your body.

16. Now spend about fifteen minutes just being with yourself and your experience. Write down your impressions of what eating like a thin person was like for you.

_____

_____

_____

_____

_____

_____

_____

_____

17. Have dinner at approximately 6:00 p.m., following the same procedure exactly, except for step 15. Instead of throwing the food away, wrap some of it up and save it for later.

18. Just before bedtime take a moment to reflect on your experience during your thin day. Congratulate yourself for letting

your thin person be in control. Then do the following exercise before going to sleep.

EXERCISE

How did you feel about working on your list of incompletions between meals today? Was it easy? fun? a chore?

_____

_____

_____

_____

In Chapter 9 we'll talk about making the choice between the Diet Mentality and the Thin Mentality. Now that you've had an opportunity to experience what it might be like for you to be thin, you'll be clearer about the choice you'll want to make. But before we reach the crossroads, I want to discuss in the next chapter why you might decide to choose fat over thin. As you'll see, the decision is not as clear-cut as it may at first appear.

CHAPTER 7

Why You Might Really Choose
Fat Over Thin

Most of us who have had a weight problem have never actually chosen to be the way we are. In our culture, there's so much emphasis on being thin that it seems to go without saying that every overweight person should want to be thin. This is where the Diet Mentality does most of its damage, with the idea that thin is good and fat is bad.

As we've already seen, people do what they do for good reasons — you choose not to go on a diet because your reasons are better than your reasons for going on a diet. By the same token, people have a weight problem for a good reason — somehow it still works better for them than being thin, or at least they think it does.

In this chapter we're going to look at why some people might prefer to be fat. If you're uncomfortable with what you discover in the following sections, don't beat yourself up. We're preparing you to make a choice, and in order for it to be an intelligent choice, you need to know as much as you can about being overweight.

Even more important, the sections in this chapter are designed to show you how your being fat is intricately tied to important aspects of your life. As we've already seen, trying to diet away the fat is not going to get the job done. You have to know the magnitude and complexity of the problem before you can decide what to do about it. The Diet Mentality has payoffs that can be very reasonable and attractive. Let's look at the major ones.

Bake Someone Happy: Parents, Spouses, Food, and You

This one is at the very heart of why you might want to choose fat over thin. Food is woven into our relationships with other people in so many ways that it boggles the mind.

Sometimes our parents use food to tell us that they love us. They can't find another way to say it, so they bake a cake or "bring home the bacon." Sometimes they use food to get us to spend time with them. Mother will put *bait* on the table just to make everyone sit down and talk to each other. Parents offer us food to show they love us, and we in turn eat the food to show that we love them.

Barbara, from Houston, wrote:

> I started getting fat when I was about thirteen years old. At that time my mother (who had been divorced for several years) was out of work and my older sisters were supporting our family. I imagine that my mother felt helpless and useless and needed to do something that would make her feel good about herself.
>
> We began a sort of ritual that year. When I would come from from school, she would already have dinner ready and would encourage me to eat. Then my sisters came home from work, and she would again encourage me to eat.
>
> Somehow I could sense how important it was to her, so I began eating two dinners every night. I wasn't her favorite child, so I was always looking for ways to get her approval. Since I could always count on her approval for eating, even for overeating, I ate the two dinners and got fat.
>
> Overeating was not what I wanted, but what mother wanted. To do what I wanted, to be thin, I would have risked her disapproval, and I would have felt disloyal to her, both of which seemed dreadful to me at the time.
>
> I realize now that I was playing a losing game with her. I wasn't doing what I wanted to do, so I wasn't satisifed. And of course I really couldn't fulfill her need

to feel useful. She still felt awful about being out of work. My mother eventually got a job and we quit the two-dinner-per-night ritual, but by that time I was already fat.

I understand now that the game we played came out of our struggle to love and be loved by one another. Knowing that makes it possible for me to forgive both myself and my mother.

EXERCISE (2 minutes)

1. "These are all the reasons I ate in order to win my parents' love or approval:"

a.

b.

c.

d.

e.

f.

It's easy to get mixed messages from parents. They want you to be attractive, and they encourage you to diet, but then they keep all this delicious food around. They say they support you in losing weight, but sometimes they act strange when you do. A woman in one of our seminars told me that she and her mother were both overweight and were always talking about diets and encouraging one another. It seemed to be the one thing they had in common. But when this woman started to lose weight and her mother didn't, they stopped speaking to one another.

Parents are sometimes pretty hard to win over. Because they love us, they want us to be as good as we can be. But as soon as we start approaching the goals they set for us, whether in sports, grades, or weight, they raise their standards. For them we can never do quite enough.

If you're trying to get thin in order to please your parents, you're fighting an uphill battle. As soon as you get close, their standards go up. They'll want something else from you, and you may never experience satisfaction in losing the weight.

That's one of the tricks we learned from our parents. We're always raising our standards and then beating ourselves up because we fail to live up to those standards. Our parents believed a good spanking would make us better, but it didn't — it just made us sneakier. The same thing happens when we beat ourselves up about our weight.

Mary shared in Houston that when she thinks about her parents, she can actually taste certain foods in her mouth. "With my mother," she said, "I can actually taste apple pie when I think about her, and I feel all warm and cozy inside. With my father, it's cabbage. He always used to make me finish my cabbage before I left the table." Food was so much a part of her relationship with her parents that she can actually taste parent memories.

EXERCISES (8 minutes)

1. "These are the foods I remember when I think about my parents:"

a.

b.

c.

d.

e.

f.

2. "These are the things my parents usually talked about at the dinner table:"

a.

b.

c.

3. "These are the general attitudes my parents gave me about my body:"

a.

b.

c.

4. "These are the circumstances in which my parents overate:"

a.

b.

c.

5. "These are the circumstances in which I overeat:"

a.

b.

c.

d.

e.

6. "These are the subtle messages I got from them about food:"

a.

b.

c.

A Few Stories About Parents and Fat

When I was about seven years old, my father came home from serving in the Navy during World War II. He was six feet tall, very strong and muscular. I was a skinny kid, and I wanted more than anything to look like my father.

I tried everything to put on weight. I saved my money until I had enough to buy a bottle of Wate-On, used it, and gained five pounds. But then as soon as the bottle ran out and before I could save the money to buy another bottle, I lost the five pounds.

Everyone said, "Don't worry. You'll grow up to look just like your dad." But I didn't want to wait. My whole life was about being like him.

When I was sixteen, I began lifting weights every day, and in three months I grew six inches and gained forty-five pounds. I was in heaven. Fourteen years later I looked just as my father had looked when he got back from the Navy. I'd done what I wanted to do and never thought about it again until I was thirty-five.

Then one day I looked in the mirror and saw my head on my father's body — not the body he had when he came home from the war, but the body he had when *he* was thirty-five.

All those years my mind had been snapping pictures of him as he grew older, and I'd continued to pattern my body after his. I even took to drinking beer the way he did, and now I had his beer-belly to show for it.

As I looked in the mirror, I realized that even though I still loved my father, I didn't have to have the same body he had. I had my own life to live, and I wanted my own body. At first I felt a terrible sadness. Then I realized I could love him without spending the rest of my life duplicating his body. I started to visualize the body I would want if there were no one else on the earth, if there were no one to compare myself with or impress. The image grew clearer and clearer to me, and that's the body I decided to have.

None of what happened was my father's fault, but it had a tremendous impact on my life. We often let our parents influence us without their even knowing it.

EXERCISES (8 minutes)

1. Get comfortable, close your eyes, and spend the next five minutes visualizing the body you would create for yourself if there were no one else on earth. When you've finished, describe it in detail.

2. Are you willing at this moment to create that body for yourself?

Yes ☐   No ☐

   People tell all kinds of stories about their relationships with parents, family, and food. Sometimes an idle comment that wasn't meant to do any harm can set up a lifetime of beliefs.

   Sarah, who lives in Oakland, told about the time one of her father's friends came over to visit. Her father welcomed him and asked if he'd like something to eat. The friend said he wasn't hungry, and her father replied, *"You have to be hungry to eat?"*

EXERCISE (3 minutes)

"These are the phrases relating to food that I remember from childhood:"

a.

b.

c.

d.

e.

Denise, who took the same seminar as Sarah, said that she was naturally thin until she was in her mid-teens. "When I was about fourteen," she said, "I noticed that my older sister, who was overweight, was getting lots of attention. She had to have special clothes, better clothes, to make her look good even though she was fat. I also wanted beautiful clothes and attention, and it wasn't long before I started putting on weight. I never realized till today that I don't have to do that anymore."

You can learn habits and beliefs very early in life. Did your mother or father use food to get you to sit down and be with them? Recall what it was like at the family dinner table. What kinds of feelings did you have?

Were you ever rewarded for eating a lot?

Did you eat to avoid punishment or to keep from having to talk about problems?

Food can be a great barrier. You can put it between you and other people to avoid any real contact. If you're both eating, it's easy for your attention to be on the food instead of on one another.

We've already talked about some of the ways a struggle with weight can affect relationships, and there are more. One is the subtle message you get from the person trying to help you lose weight that you aren't OK the way you are. That's not a very nice feeling to live with. If you're receiving that message, consciously or unconsciously, you're probably going to feel some resentment. You'll get them back somehow, with the weight or with some other weapon.

Another game you can play with parents or your spouse or anyone else close to you is the game of, "Even if I lose weight, I know you'll never praise or acknowledge me enough, or in the right way." Guess what? You're probably right. Most people aren't mind-readers. They don't know how you want them to acknowledge you unless you tell them.

Sometimes we don't tell people what we want because we're afraid they won't want to give it to us or because they'll think we're terrible for asking. That's the chance we take. They may think just that. But at least you've given them all the information they need to support you. If they don't want to do it, that's their choice and that tells you something about your relationship with them. The more you're able to love and accept yourself, the easier it will be for people around you to do the same.

Maybe human beings, like automobiles, should have owners' manuals to tell others how they work. There should be a book that tells us what to say and how and when to say it to one another. As it is, however, if we want something from another person — support, acknowledgment, love, encouragement — we have to tell them exactly what it is.

You can sit around hoping, wishing, or praying that they'll do the right thing, but that doesn't usually get you anywhere. If you and I are sitting in a room together, and I start thinking it would be so nice if you'd get me a cup of coffee, then I'd better tell you about it. Otherwise, I might sit there the whole afternoon wondering why you hadn't thought of it yourself.

A man named Sam told us in the Los Angeles seminar how he got his mother to support him. Every year when he would go home for Christmas, she would have the refrigerator and the freezer stuffed with food he loved. If he ever said he liked anything, he could count on it being there when he got home. He would usually come back weighing ten pounds more than he did when he left.

One year he called his mother before he went home and told her he didn't want to do that to himself again this year. He explained that he loved her and her food, but that eating the way he usually did when he went home made him unhappy in the long run. She understood and cooked sensible meals for him. Sam got the food that he wanted, and his mother got to support him, which was really what she wanted to do.

EXERCISES (5 minutes)

1. What specific things do you want in the way of support from the people in your life?

a.

b.

c.

d.

e.

2. Whom do you need to tell?

a.

b.

c.

d.

e.

3. When are you going to tell them? "By_____(date) I
will have told everyone I need to tell exactly what I want from them
in the way of support."

Fat and Sex

I'm always amazed at the number of times this subject comes up
at the Diets Don't Work Seminar. We start out talking about
weight, and usually by the middle of the afternoon we're talking
about sex. It's almost impossible to talk about weight, it seems,
without also talking about sex and relationships. There is a link
between the two.

Many people come right out and say that one reason they keep
their weight on is because they don't want to confront the whole
issue of sex and relationships. It isn't any big revelation to them;
they know exactly what they're doing, it's part of the plan.

Some of them have been hurt badly in relationships and will do anything to avoid becoming involved in one again. They figure weight is a foolproof method — no one wants you when you're fat, they reason. It's a subtle way to avoid relationships without wearing a sign that says, "Don't come near me."

It can be embarrassing to say you don't want to have a relationship. Everybody should want to have one, right? But these people have been burned, and they don't want to be burned again. If you got mugged every time you wore a red dress, how long would you continue to wear red dresses?

They have it in their mind that if they're thin, they will automatically have a relationship. That's part of the fantasy of being thin, but it's not necessarily the reality. Ask some thin people about it. They'll tell you that being thin is no guarantee of having a relationship or of having the kind of relationship you want.

Sometimes, people who want to avoid relationships haven't even been burned. For some reason, they just don't want to get involved with another person or with sex. Maybe they don't know exactly what that reason is, but they do know they don't want to get mixed up in the sexual arena. They figure the best way to do that is to keep themselves from being attractive. (They don't always succeed in being unattractive, by the way, even if they are overweight. There are some people who think fat is sexy. They like their mates to be soft and cuddly. In some cultures, fatness is a sign of beauty.)

Even if someone is attracted to them despite their weight, they can always fall back on the old Woody Allen saying, "I would never join a club that would have me as a member." "If the guy is attracted to someone as fat and unattractive as I am," they reason, "he must be a creep."

Another way people connect sex and weight is through their lover or spouse. If they were to become thin and were attractive to other people, it would be threatening to their spouse. He or she would turn all squirrelly on them. Even worse, if other relationships were available to them, they might just jump at the opportunity. They don't trust themselves not to do this. Who knows what would happen if they suddenly became available and entered the sexual marketplace?

As long as they're overweight, they don't have to deal with the problem at all. They can maintain the status quo because no one else is going to be attracted to them anyway. It doesn't threaten their spouse, and it doesn't threaten them. If you don't have a choice, you can't make the wrong decision and ruin your present relationship.

For some people the struggle with weight has become an integral part of their intimate relationships. Often the spouse wants them to lose weight and is always giving them advice about how to do it, badgering them to go on a diet, and "supporting" them by teasing, manipulating, punishing, and goading them. Overweight people don't usually enjoy such treatment, but the issue takes up such a large part of their relationship that they may wonder how they would fill the void if it were gone. If they didn't have the issue of weight to talk and argue about, what would they say to each other?

Sometimes a spouse inadvertently becomes a party to the Diet Mentality. Whether or not he says it out loud, a husband, for example, may get the message across that if the weight doesn't go away, then he will. He holds that like an axe over his wife's head and uses it to manipulate her. If she can't lose weight, she can at least do a better job on his shirts, or come with him to a party she doesn't want to go to, or do something else to make up for being fat.

Just try to lose weight with that hanging over your head. It's human nature to resist anything you have to do and haven't chosen for yourself. The resistance might not be conscious, but it's there. Who wants to be a kid again? To be powerless and have to do what others tell you to do? You'll fight them to the death, even if "they" are your employer or spouse, and even if you say you want the results it will produce.

Most people don't mean to be unsupportive. Even some doctors have been taught that the way to help people lose weight is to give them a hard time about being fat. They're not necessarily trying to make you feel terrible; they just want to help and don't know how.

I've been talking so far about the woman who's fat, but it can just as easily be the other way around. It can be the man who's overweight, and the woman who's trying to get him to lose. In either case some part of the relationship turns into a battle of manipulation.

In most cases neither party really knows what they want or what the other person wants. The spouse may say he wants you to lose weight but may really be afraid that if you do, he'll have some competition. So he sabotages you, takes you out to dinner in a fancy restaurant. Or you may say you really do want to lose, but are afraid of what you'll do with the new freedom. Or you might not want to lose the leverage you have over him by your ability to gain or lose weight. You can punish him by gaining and reward him by losing. He can't do anything about it because you have all the cards.

Another battle cry is, "I don't want to be loved only for my body." By staying fat you can test the other person to see if he loves you for your body or for who you really are. Probably he does appreciate you as you are, or he wouldn't put up with the weight. Look and see whom you're really testing. Could it be yourself?

Some women are afraid that if they lose weight, their breasts will get smaller or they won't have any hips. Both men and women are sometimes afraid they won't have their weight to throw around anymore. We may have been told, "I love you because there's so much of you to love," and we may have believed it. We may believe that if we lose the weight, we will become even more unattractive.

I've often heard people describe their perfect weight as their *hunting weight.* If they were that size, they say, they would be out there on the prowl. Then God knows what would happen — they might be besieged with offers and would have to make some choices. Members of the opposite sex might be clawing at their body. There would be no rest. Sometimes this sounds great, but at other times it just sounds like a new set of problems. The familiar patterns are usually a lot more comfortable, especially if you've gotten hurt or rejected while you were out there hunting.

EXERCISES (3 minutes)

1. "These are the ways being overweight influences how I approach sex and relationships:"

a.

b.

c.

d.

e.

2. "These are the payoffs I get for having my weight be an obstacle to relationships:"

a.

b.

c.

d.

e.

Fat and Power?

Often it seems like being overweight isn't about fat at all, but about power. Strange as it may seem, you wield a lot of control over others by being fat. People worry about you. They cajole you. They want to help you. They give you attention. even if it means getting angry with you and goading you.

Attention is something that people want very badly. Have you ever noticed how children use their behavior to get attention? Children are experts at this. Any time you give them attention for doing something, they'll tend to do it again. If you give them more attention for making trouble than for cleaning up their room, they're very likely to make more trouble. Even punishment is a form of attention. If they get negative attention for being bad, they'll be bad. If they get positive attention for being good, they'll be good.

If you're getting more attention for being overweight than you did for being thin, the chances are that you will continue to be overweight. This holds true whether the attention is from yourself or from others. If you give yourself a lot of attention for your fat, if you're always thinking and worrying about it, then you're getting something out of being overweight that you might not get if you were thin.

If you're engaged in a struggle with someone over your weight, you're getting attention and have the power to manipulate them. You can make them happy or miserable just by whether or not you eat that Sara Lee coffeecake.

You can actually bind people to you by being fat. Maybe you're their project — they won't rest until you're thin. They love you and worry about you more because you have this problem. Maybe lots of your friends are also overweight, and your mutual struggle with fat binds you. If you lost the weight, they might go away. And well they might, if that's what your friendship is based on. But if the bond is deeper, they'll still be your friends.

Another way people connect weight and power is by actual size. Again and again we hear in the Diets Don't Work Seminar, "If I lost weight, I would feel like I might just blow away in the wind. I would feel so fragile and vulnerable. I don't like the way I look now, but at least I'm *there!*" Over the years people start to think that the presence they project into the world is related to their physical size. Somehow their weight protects them. No one is going to mess with someone that big. They're present, and everyone knows it. They can't be ignored or taken lightly. They're afraid that if they were thin, they would get pushed around, or even worse, no one would notice them.

Other people relate fat and power in just the opposite way. They're afraid of the power they think will come to them if they get thin. If they were thin, they wouldn't have any excuse for feeling powerless. They would have to get out there and become everything they've always wanted to be — sexy, powerful, and successful. The truth is, they're afraid they might not succeed. It sounds like quite a challenge, doesn't it?

What if something drastic happened in your life, and overnight you had to become exactly the person you've always wanted to be. You didn't have any choice, and you couldn't take it slowly — you had to do it all now. Part of you would probably be excited, but another part of you would be scared to face such an immense challenge so suddenly. That's how some people feel about losing their weight. They think too much would be expected of them, not only by other people, but also by themselves. Better just to go back to bed or have another cookie.

Other people have the idea that if they lost weight, they would also lose control of their lives. Things aren't so great now, but they have a tried and tested method of dealing with discomfort, stress, and anxiety — eat. What if they didn't have that? What if they had no way of regulating their emotions the way they do with food? It would be like being set adrift in a small boat in the middle of the ocean — they wouldn't know where to turn or what to do. Now at least they have something that they know works. It might not get them what they want, but at least it's familiar.

Power can play an important part in being overweight. Fear of losing it, and fear of having it, can keep the pounds on as surely as a diet.

EXERCISES (5 minutes)

1. "These are all the ways I get attention from other people for being fat:"

a.

b.

c.

d.

e.

2. "These are all the ways I get more attention from myself for being fat than I would if I were thin:"

a.

b.

c.

d.

e.

Thank you for doing these exercises. Just a little more now and you'll be through one of the most uncomfortable sections.

Fat and Success?

There are subtle differences between the ways people relate fat to power and the ways they relate fat to success. Relating fat and power usually has to do with your relationships with other people. Relating fat and success, more often than not, has to do with your relationship with yourself.

Most people think that they would be more successful if they were thin. Whether they define success in terms of career, family, relationships, or the way they feel about themselves, it's all the same. Thin equals successful. As long as they have the fat they will allow themselves to only be partially successful. But they're sure they would be even more successful if they were thin.

The fear of success is by no means unique to people who are overweight. Thin people just use other means to keep themselves from being wholly successful. Why are we afraid of success? There are many reasons, even some good ones. It's a complicated issue, and much has been written about it. Here we'll only deal with how the fear of success can prevent you from losing weight.

Some people fear success because they think if they had everything they wanted, their lives would be over. What would you do once you had everything? You would have nothing to occupy your time, no more problems to solve, nothing to care about. What would you do with all the energy you'd learned to use getting to be where you are? What would be the point in living?

Let me tell you a secret: you can always come up with a new problem. It's human nature to create problems and solve them; we do it instinctively. That's how we learn and grow. If you talk to a person who is fabulously rich, fabulously thin, and fabulously happy, you'll probably discover that there's some new problem that he or she is working on. That level of success brings its own problems.

Also, every solution you come up with can be counted on to generate your next problem. Maybe now that you have this great new car, you have to find a mechanic who will treat it like his own. Or you've found the person of your dreams and can't decide whether to honeymoon on Galveston Island or in Miami? There's always going to be some new challenge to face, something exciting on the horizon. Trust it. Ask anyone you think is successful.

Another thing people fear about success is that they won't blend into the crowd anymore, others will notice them and recognize that they have what it takes to get what they want. And they're afraid they won't live up to those expectations.

Maybe you think others will be watching you and won't ever let you fail again. Everyone will know if you have a relationship that doesn't turn out perfectly, or if you sneak into Baskin-Robbins for a mini-binge. Your life will be in the spotlight, and you'll never again be able to commit those secret little indiscretions. Or people may become jealous of you. If you've ever been envious of someone who's successful, then you can't help thinking that people are going to feel the same way toward you. You *know* all the backbiting and faultfinding that goes on. You might find yourself rejected and alone, and that's not what you want.

In addition, you don't know what you would be like if you were successful. Maybe you would become nasty and overbearing. Maybe success wouldn't look so good on you. At least now your situation is familiar, you know who you are. To become a completely new person is frightening.

Some people play just the opposite game. They want to prove that they can be successful despite their fat. According to a recent study, ten pounds can make the difference between getting and not getting a job, between getting and not getting a promotion. But these people want to show the world that they can make it anyway. They can't seem to prove often enough that their worth, value, and abilities aren't determined by their weight.

Other people keep their weight because they think they should be judged on their abilities but haven't been. If the world's criterion for success is being thin, they conclude, they're going to protest against it. They won't lose weight just to get a job or promotion. They would rather be right than thin.

EXERCISES (10 minutes)

1. "These are all the ways I use being overweight to keep from being completely successful:"

a.

b.

c.

d.

e.

2. "These are the new problems I would like to exchange for the problem of being overweight:"

a.

b.

c.

d.

e.

3. "These are the reasons I fear becoming more visible:"

a.

b.

c.

d.

e.

4. "This is how being overweight influences my relationships with:"

Sex

Power

Success

5. "I think I'm overweight because:"

a.

b.

c.

d.

e.

6. "These are a few more reasons I have for overeating:"

a.

b.

c.

d.

e.

There may be times when you prefer the payoffs of being fat to the benefits of being thin. If you do, that's OK; you get to choose. But recognize that in the process you lose the joy that the thin person can bring to your life.

The Person in the Mirror

Another reason you might choose fat over thin is that you would have to change your self-image to be thin, and that seems hard, even impossible. For a long time you've thought of yourself as a certain kind of person. Now if you want to be thin, you're going to have to let go of that image and create another. The old person, the fat person inside you, isn't going to like that. You'd better be prepared for some resistance.

In a way it's a kind of death. There may be the same kind of sadness that I experienced when I let go of my father. You don't particularly like the old friend you see in the mirror, but sometimes old friendships die hard, even though you don't really want them to continue, and they don't support you where you are now.

You have to recognize that and focus on the positive. Focus on the new person, the thin person, that is emerging as a replacement. That person is a lot happier and probably closer to who you really are. That new, thin person is going to carry you to a whole new level of being.

Imagine you're trading in an old, beaten-up station wagon for a spiffy little sports car. If you've had the station wagon for a long time, you may experience some sadness in giving it up. But in the end, since you want the sports car, you just have to say goodbye to the station wagon, thank it for all the pleasure it has given you, and focus on enjoying your new car.

But What If...

It's easy to convince people to adopt the first, third, and fourth guidelines of eating like a thin person: eating only when you're hungry, stopping when your body has had enough, and not eating on automatic. The guideline that's scary to them is the second guideline, eating exactly what you want to eat.

Most people are afraid they'll gain pounds by the score during the first few weeks. The thought of letting yourself go and giving yourself permission to eat what you want is terrifying. It goes against everything in the Diet Mentality. You may assume you'll want to eat nothing but Ho-Hos, cupcakes, lasagna, and cream pies. You see, anything you think you can't have takes on an aura of forbiddenness and desirability; you believe you're going to want it all the time. But if you give yourself permission to have it, that insatiable desire fades away.

Giving yourself that permission eliminates what I call Last Supper eating. How many times have you looked down at a bag of brownies and thought they would be your last? Or *should* be your last? Those brownies become very special to you. You're a condemned person, and this is your last fling. Brownies become the most fascinating and succulent of foods. So when you fantasize about food, brownies are bound to be in the picture. If you could have a brownie anytime you wanted one, what would be the big deal?

A week after the Diets Don't Work Seminar in Los Angeles, Ellen told us, "The strange thing was that I'd always thought if I could really eat anything I wanted, I would pig out on candy and shakes. I tried it, but something was different now. They didn't taste the way I thought they would."

Your body is not dumb. It has instincts for self-preservation. It also has instincts for health and happiness. All the rules and deprivations you've been using only get in the way of those instincts.

Noreen, who lives in Aspen, said, "The first day I let myself have five Milky Ways. My mother never let me eat them when I was a child, and I guess I had always thought of them as the most forbidden of forbidden fruit. It was funny, because the next day I was grocery shopping and when I got to the candy section and my eyes fell on those Milky Ways, I couldn't stand the sight of them. My body was starting to assert a life of its own. The food it wanted that day was carrots, so off I went to the vegetable section."

When you're riding a horse up and down a steep trail, sometimes it's best just to give the horse its head. You let him pick the path, rather than trying to tell him where to go. The horse's instincts are better than yours, and so are your body's.

You don't have to force your body to eat things it doesn't want. You may buy a whole refrigerator full of carrots and celery, but your body may peek inside and say, "Yuk! I want a hamburger." That's probably because it needs a hamburger.

How many times have you bought a refrigerator full of "thin food" and watched it rot? There's a whole generation of children growing up now who think that diet cottage cheese is something you bring home from the store, put in the refrigerator, let spoil, and then throw away.

Your body knows. Christine, who lives in San Francisco, said that for a week she found herself craving raisins and parsley. She didn't understand why, but she couldn't get enough of either of them. "What an odd combination," she thought. Then someone told her that they were both high in iron. Her body was screaming at her to give it iron, and its message manifested in what she was craving.

When you get used to eating like this, your body starts to send you messages. It will tell you what it wants and what it needs. It doesn't have any axes to grind other than its own well-being. It doesn't have any of the attitudes and patterns and points of view that you do. It only knows what's going to make it strong and healthy. Let it speak to you. Trust that your body is on your side and has your best interests at heart.

EXERCISES (6 minutes)

1. "These are my worst fears about what would happen if I gave myself permission to eat whatever I wanted:"

a.

b.

c.

d.

e.

2. "These are the best things that could happen if I gave myself permission to eat whatever I wanted:"

a.

b.

c.

d.

e.

3. "I can trust my body's instincts because:"

a.

b.

c.

d.

e.

The Fat Person's Tactics

The two persons inside you, the fat person and the thin person, are at odds. They operate in different ways, and they want different things. The same world isn't going to work for both of them.

The first thing you have to recognize is that the fat person has the edge right now. He's bigger, stronger, more clever, and more devious. He's been getting all the attention. You've been feeding him while you starved the thin person. The fat person has a lot of influence over your behavior right now. When you start to replace him with the thin person, he's going to put up a fight. He's going to try to make you as uncomfortable as he can.

The fat person is more devious than you can possibly imagine. The more threatened he gets, the more desperate and devious he becomes. He's starting to slip off the ledge and his fingernails are clawing at your throat.

He may try to fool you into thinking he's on your side. He may have been sitting on your shoulder while you've been reading this book, solemnly nodding his head and agreeing with everything that's been said. But when push comes to shove, he's going to use that very information against you.

This is when he starts coming up with the "Yeah, but's..." Good! These are his last-ditch efforts.

- "Yeah, but no one can change themselves and start thinking that differently from the way they have in the past."
- "Yeah, but this is just somebody trying to kid you into trying again and failing. Just because *they* did it doesn't mean *you* can."
- "Yeah, but if it were really that easy, everyone would have done it by now."
- "Yeah, but I'm okay just the way I am. Looks aren't that important to me."
- "Yeah, but look at all the trouble you would get into if you lost weight. You couldn't hide, and you would be threatening to other people. Things aren't so bad the way they are now."
- "Yeah, but I don't have what it takes to change."
- "Yeah, but I give so much to other people, and eating is the only thing I give to myself."

A woman named Patty, from San Francisco, shared that she'd found a great way of dealing with those voices. She treated them the same way she did her children. Every day her son would come home and tell her the latest thing he'd decided to be when he grew up. One day he would say, "Mommy, I'm going to be an astronaut." The next day he would come home and say, "Mommy, guess what! I'm going to be an engineer!" She would just smile and nod her head. She wouldn't try to fight with him or reason with him, and she didn't take anything he said too seriously.

That's how Patty started treating the voices. She would just smile, nod her head, and not believe a word of it. She knew that's just how voices are. You don't have to take what they say to heart.

The fat person inside you wants desperately to persuade you that you don't really want to be attractive in the end, that you don't want to give up your individuality and invisibility and expose yourself to change, that you want an excuse to hide and play the game of life for small stakes. He doesn't want you to find out that you have a purpose in life other than trying to lose weight. And he doesn't want you to encounter anything new and exciting.

He tries to convince you that you won't be able to handle new challenges. He reminds you that if you lost your weight, you wouldn't have anything to complain about. He says, "Who do you think you are?" and tries to make you think it's egotistical to have your body exactly the way you want it to be. He wants to keep things just the way they are.

The way things are now, you see, he's in the center stage, he has all the attention. And he knows if you start listening to the thin person inside you, his game will be over.

You don't have to let the fat person get to you, though. You have a weapon he doesn't know about, and it can cut through just about anything: you know his game plan. You know how he operates. You know the tricks he will try to use on you, and you can head him off before he gets started.

You have something even better than that. You have detachment. You can watch him rant and rave and scream as if you were watching a movie, and not get sucked in. You can wait out the storm, knowing that the way he acts doesn't have to upset you. You can stand firm, knowing that you're not going to beat yourself up for what he's doing. You just wait, watch, and provide a nurturing environment for the thin person.

Just remember that the fat person isn't you. Any time you play into his game, any time you give him energy and attention, he gains strength. And any time you just watch with detachment, you weaken him. The weaker he gets, the stronger the thin person becomes.

EXERCISES (5 minutes)

1. "These are the phrases that the fat person inside me whispers — or yells — in my ear:"

a.

b.

c.

d.

e.

2. "These are the best ways for me to combat those voices when I hear them:"

a.

b.

c.

d.

e.

The Fat Person's Trump Card

If you play bridge, you know that trump cards are the cards you reserve till the end of the game, when nothing else will work. What trump cards do you suppose the fat person inside you is holding? It's getting down to the wire. You're about to choose between fat and thin, and you've already deprived him of most of the old tricks he's been using on you. You're starting to understand how he plays. That puts him at a disadvantage, and he knows it. He's going to have to make a final stand, something that's sure to lure you back to him. What do you suppose it will be?

The fat person inside you has something in his arsenal we haven't discussed yet. I learned about it from a man named Stewart Emery of Actualizations, and it's the fat person's last resort. Actually it's so subtle and so pervasive hardly anyone ever notices.

As babies we have to figure out the best way to get attention, right? And as it turns out, just about the most effective way to get attention, aside from yelling and screaming, is to do something that pleases other people. If we smile at Mommy and Daddy, for instance, that makes them ecstatic, and they call everyone else over to take a look at us. Please them, earn their approval, and we get all the attention we want.

Then one day the old trick doesn't work anymore. Say we've been drawing pictures with crayons and the folks have been loving it. So we decide to take Mommy's brushes and paints and draw a big picture all over the living room wall. Won't they be pleased!

But when they come home, instead of admiring our masterpiece, they scream at us, give us a whomp on the rump, and send us to bed without supper. "Wait a minute!" we think. "What went wrong?" — our first major failure to win approval.

After this happens a few times more, we make a decision about ourselves: *"I can't win!"* Then the question becomes how to avoid losing. And the answer is simple — play small. Don't try to win, don't play 100%. Hold back and maybe they won't notice us. Do as little as possible, don't ever put ourselves on the line. That decision influences how we act for the rest of our lives, and we wind up playing for matchsticks in a world of abundance.

That's the fat person's trump card, and for some people weight is the perfect excuse. If you weren't overweight and could get on with the rest of your life, you might fail. This way you're safe. It's a subtle maneuver, difficult to pin down, but as any bridge player will tell you, you have a better chance of winning if you know the other person's cards.

EXERCISES (3 minutes)

1. "These are the ways I play the game of life for small stakes:"

a.

b.

c.

d.

e.

2. "These are the ways I hold myself back in order to avoid failing:"

a.

b.

c.

d.

e.

At the Crossroads

So now you have a pretty good idea of why being overweight can be attractive. It's not so crazy to be fat, even to choose consciously to be fat. By now you've also gotten an idea of what it might be like for you to develop the Thin Mentality we discussed in Chapter 7. And of course you're well-acquainted with the Diet Mentality. You're at the crossroads. In the next chapter you'll make the big decision.

Before we get there, I want you to know that none of the choices is any better or easier or more right than the others. There's only the choice that's appropriate for you. All you have to do now is tell the truth.

CHAPTER 8

Making the Choice

At last we've arrived at the moment of truth. Tomorrow is the beginning of the rest of your life. You have four choices. As you read through them, you'll know the one that's right for you, and it may not be the one you had in mind when you started this book. Whatever your choice, do it affirmatively. Choose it, accept it, and give it all of your support. Ready? Here goes.

Fat and Unhappy

This is the choice of the Diet Mentality. All you have to do is continue what you've been doing. Continue on the diet/binge rollercoaster. Continue to beat yourself up about your weight, your inability to stick to a diet. Deprive yourself and restrict your activities and relationships because of your weight. Worry as much as possible about how much you weigh, what you're eating or not eating. Tell yourself constantly what a failure you are. And above all, keep trying every new diet that comes out. You're already an expert at this, so there's no need to elaborate further.

The important part of this option is acknowledging that you want to be unhappy. Most of us say that we want to be happy, but as we've seen, there are a lot of advantages to being unhappy. We get attention, we get sympathy, we have excuses, people fuss over us and try to help us. If this is truly what you want, it's extremely important to be honest about it. People who say they want to be happy and really don't are going to be constantly at odds with themselves.

Take a minute to see if there's anything you're getting out of being unhappy that you wouldn't get if you were happy. For example, Jan, who lives in Los Angeles, shared after the seminar that her frequent periods of depression had disappeared. She realized, she said, that she had been using them to get attention from her husband. Whenever she was depressed, she noticed, he came home early for dinner. When she felt good, he often had business dinners or worked late. She was getting something out of being unhappy that she didn't get when she was happy. In this case Jan decided she wanted to be happy, so she gave up her depressions. As a result, her husband started coming home early more often.

To get clear in your mind about where you stand with this option, do the following exercise.

EXERCISE (3 minutes)

"These are the benefits I get out of being unhappy:"

a.

b.

c.

d.

e.

Would you be willing to give these benefits up in order to be happy?

Thin and Miserable

It's just like fat and unhappy except that you spend 98% of your energy and time staying thin by effort, struggle, and diets.

Fat and Happy

Fat and happy? You must think I'm kidding. Who could be fat and happy? The two don't go together. Let's take a look.

Given everything that you've done so far to lose weight and everything you're willing to do (or not willing to do) from now on, the truth may actually be that you are never going to get thin. If that's the case, then wouldn't the most practical thing be to accept yourself the way you are and get on with your life? If deep in your heart you know you really aren't willing to do what's necessary to be thin, then the most sensible, practical, and loving thing you can do for yourself is to accept yourself the way you are. Quit all this beating yourself up about your weight, and use that energy to start living the way you want to.

Let's suppose you had a friend who was thirty-five years old and five feet two. All his life he'd wanted to be seven feet tall. He'd gone on all the tall diets, done all the tall exercises, bought tall clothes hoping he would grow into them. He went to doctors, meditated, hoped, prayed, but he never grew. Every day he just became more miserable because he wasn't growing.

As his friend, wouldn't you tell him to let go of the idea of being seven feet tall and accept himself the way he was so he could be happy? What if it's the same with weight? What if some people are just fat and others are just thin? What if there really is no solution? What would you do? Would you keep torturing yourself for the rest of your life? You may feel that this is impossible because everybody knows it's bad to be fat. But what if that's a decision you can change? Maybe you can just accept being overweight as a neutral fact about you, like having brown hair or hazel eyes. What if fat were just fat?

Think of all the things you could do if you just gave up and enjoyed being the way you are. You'd never again have to worry about dieting. You could buy clothes that were comfortable, rather than buying them one size too small to try to look smaller than you are. You could eat whatever you wanted and enjoy it. You could lean back and laugh when people bought diet books. You could stop putting your life on hold until after you were thin and start living it fully right now.

Again and again people have told us that the very act of getting off their own backs about losing weight allowed them to lose it. Elaine, from Aspen, said, "I couldn't believe what happened when I decided to be fat and happy. It was as if there was nothing to fight against with food, so I lost interest. One day I even forgot to eat till dinner. Me, who used to eat at least five meals a day! Since there was no more battle, eating became rather dull."

It's a great blow to the Diet Mentality when you accept yourself exactly the way you are. Things just naturally start to turn around. Part of it is that if you start caring enough about yourself to get off your own back, you eliminate many of your reasons for overeating.

Carol, who lives in San Francisco, is thirty-five and has been naturally thin for twenty years. But when she was fourteen, she weighed 145, twenty pounds more than she does now.

> I was in high school and just miserable. Everything in my life revolved around food — what I was eating, what I wasn't eating, what I was going to eat. It was as if there was a demon inside me that wouldn't let me stop thinking about my weight.
>
> Back then, there wasn't as much information about diets as there is now, but I had this instinctive sense that they wouldn't work for me. I knew that even on the off-chance I could stick to one until I lost weight, it would be like living in chains, and I would still hate myself.
>
> I didn't understand the Diet Mentality, but I was a smart kid. I figured out that I had two problems: one was that I was fat, and the other was that I was always worried about being fat. I figured that I could eliminate

50% of my problems overnight just by not worrying about it anymore.

At first I thought, "You can't give in like that. It would be like settling for second best. Surely you're a better person than that." It was quite a blow to my ego. It took a lot of humility to accept myself the way I was, but I was so miserable I would have done anything. I stopped trying to stuff myself into size 12s and went out and bought a size 14 skirt. I let myself eat what I wanted and just stopped worrying about it.

I don't know how I did it. Maybe there's no how. I just stopped. Every time the voices in my head started screaming, I would remind them that it was OK for me to be the way I am.

Then a funny thing started happening — I started losing weight. My mother became worried and took me to the doctor. She thought I had cancer. He said I was in great shape, and I continued to lose. After a month I was down to 125, and I've stayed that way ever since, eating whatever I've wanted.

The results of choosing this option aren't always as dramatic, but one fact remains: you don't have a prayer of changing anything about yourself until you accept it exactly the way it is. If you're running away from it, denying it, covering it up, then it's in control.

You see, we tend to think that happiness comes from outside us — from our circumstances, from other people, from material things, from reaching our goals. But the exact opposite is true; happiness comes from within. We bring the happiness to our circumstances, our relationships, our goals, our lives. Things, achievements, other people, can never make us happy. If they could, there wouldn't be so many miserable people who are rich or successful or involved in a relationship.

There's an old saying, "Success is getting what you want; happiness is wanting what you get." You can be happy instantly by wanting what you already have. To be miserable all you have to do is want what you don't have. You see, at some point in your life, you did want what you now have. For instance, sometime in the past you decided that you wanted to overeat more than you wanted to be thin and you can lighten up about the whole situation by acknowledging that as the truth. Of course, now you may want to have a thin body, but you'll never be happy if you can't accept your situation as it is right now.

It takes a lot of courage to choose this option. It goes against everything written or spoken in our culture on the subject of weight. But you can end weight as a problem in your life forever in one instant just by choosing this option. To assist you in getting clear about this, please do the following exercise.

EXERCISES (5 minutes)

1. "These are the advantages I foresee for myself in giving myself permission to be fat and happy:"

a.

b.

c.

2. "These are the disadvantages I foresee for myself in giving myself permission to be fat and happy:"

a.

b.

c.

3 "If I accepted myself just the way I am and gave myself permission to get on with my life, I would start doing things like:"

a.

b.

c.

d.

Thin and Happy

The fourth option you have is to let the thin person inside you come forth and take control. Just as there are a lot of fat people walking around in thin bodies, there are a lot of thin people walking around in fat bodies. If this is the case for you, if deep in your heart you know that the person inside you is really a thin person dying to get out, then you have your work cut out for you — nothing less than changing your whole attitude about your body, food, and life in general.

It requires a commitment to doing whatever is necessary to be thin and happy. It's that simple and that difficult. There are no magic wands or overnight solutions, at least not yet. If there were a diet or a magic formula, there wouldn't be any need for books like this. Everyone would be already thin.

Just as being fat and happy depends on accepting things the way they are, being thin and happy begins with acknowledging that you got fat for good reasons, you've kept the fat around for good reasons, and now you're going to forgive yourself for your past and move forward.

Choosing to be thin and happy is a journey into the unknown that's both exciting and scary. It's like changing from a smoker into a nonsmoker. In one instant you change. You make a commitment to a new way of life, with the understanding that it will bring with it a new set of problems, but also a new set of joys and rewards.

Part III of this book is devoted to supporting those of you who choose this option. We'll go into more detail there about the Thin Mentality, about how to think like a thin person. I could try telling you in advance what it will be like, but just as your weight problem is unique, evolving your thin body will also be unique. You'll need to have the courage to rely on yourself, to take your directions from inside yourself rather than from others, to be willing to make mistakes as you discover your own answers.

Letting Go

Now you've seen the four options available to you; the time has come to make the choice. In order to be totally clear about what you want, fill in the appropriate blank.

1.____ I choose to be fat and unhappy.
2.____ I choose to be thin and unhappy.
3.____ I choose to be fat and happy.
4.____ I choose to be thin and happy.

Congratulations! You've just made one of the most difficult choices you'll ever make in your life. Whatever you chose, I applaud you for your willingness to take responsibility for your weight and to do what is appropriate for you.

To complete the choosing process, the only thing left now is for you to let go of all the other possibilities and move forward affirmatively in the direction you've chosen. To illustrate what I mean by letting to, let me tell you the story of Frank "Bring 'em Back Alive" Buck, who trapped live animals for the circus.

Buck had a very interesting way of catching monkeys. He would take a coconut shell and drill two holes in it, one the size of one finger, the other the size of two fingers. Then he would tie the coconut to a tree, stuff some wild rice into it, and leave.

When he came back several hours later, he would invariably find a monkey with both hands stuck inside the coconut. The monkey's empty hands were just big enough to fit in the larger hole, but when the monkey was holding fistfuls of rice, he couldn't pull his hands out again. Even when he saw Buck coming, he wouldn't let go of the rice.

Buck would just throw a burlap bag over the monkey, take him back to the camp, and shake him out into a cage. The monkey would tumble out, still holding onto the wild rice, his hands still stuck inside the coconut. Buck would have to break the coconut open with a hammer so the monkey could get his hands out. Then the monkey would stuff the rice into his mouth, only to realize too late that he'd just sacrificed the most precious thing in the world — his freedom.

When you make a choice, any choice, you're always giving up other options; you can't have them all. The monkey couldn't have the wild rice and his freedom at the same time — he made a choice. Your choice now involves letting go of the past. Let go and go forward, regardless of the option you picked. Just let go.

From now on we're going to be talking about the thin life. (If you've chosen one of the first three options, there's really no reason for you to continue reading.) Read on, and I'll share with you some of the things I've learned about thinking, living, and eating as a thin person.

Part III
The Thin Life

CHAPTER 9

Your Breakthrough

What is a Breakthrough?

When a breakthrough happens, you begin to look at life in a new way. It's a jump into a new way of perceiving what's around you, as if you'd taken off blinders and saw a different world from the one you saw before.

A breakthrough puts you into a different state of being and alters your approach to life. You may see the same people and things around you, but you see them in a completely new way.

You've probably had several breakthroughs in your life — when you had a child, for example, or when you fell in love, or when someone close to you died. You may have had a breakthrough when you first moved away from home, or when you stopped smoking, or when you got a new job.

Helen, who lives in Los Angeles, said, "Mine came at the moment in the seminar when I realized that I was the one who was in charge of my body. I realized that I was at the end of the line, and if I kept waiting for someone or something else to do it for me, then it was never going to happen. I just gave up on everyone and everything and reached a point of hopelessness. The next thing I knew, I really was in charge!"

Breakthroughs don't always happen by chance. You can actually set out to have one. I know several people who knew they had a lot of unexpressed anger bottled up inside them and deliberately set out to pull the cork. They set up a safe environment, with someone there to watch over them, and then let it fly, sometimes for the first time in their lives. After that anger was released, they felt as if they were looking at the world through new eyes. Something had shifted inside them that made everything look different.

Breakthrough is what this book is all about — your breakthrough into being a thin person and seeing everything around you from that perspective. It's a shift that will take place inside you. It may have happened already, even without your knowing it. Just in the act of reading this book and doing the exercises, that transformation may already have taken place.

Suddenly Thin

When I see people in my seminars making their commitment to being thin and happy, it reminds me of a story that illustrates the feeling of jumping into something. A friend of mine was working on his Ph.D. at a prestigious university, and all the time he was a student, the professors treated him like a hopeless imbecile. Then when graduation day came and he was handed his diploma, suddenly those same professors started treating him like an equal, a colleague. It made him uncomfortable, because he'd gotten so used to having them treat him like a fool that he didn't quite know how to act. One minute he was a nobody, the next they were calling him Doctor.

It's like quitting smoking. One minute you're a smoker, doing all the things smokers do. Then suddenly you're a nonsmoker. At first you have to get oriented, you have to give yourself some time to discover what your special problems are going to be and how to deal with them. People are going to treat you differently. These same principles are at work when you break through to the Thin Mentality.

Doing It for You

One of the major obstacles people encounter in losing weight is that they're trying to do it to please someone else. It might be their spouse, their friends, their boss, or their children. There are many reasons for trying to lose weight to please other people, but they all have one thing in common — they don't work.

One reason they don't work is that you lose control of the game. If other people are your motivation for losing weight, then one way or another you're going to be dependent on what they say or do. You never know when a roadblock is going to fall in your path, because you can't control their actions. It also sets up an excuse for not winning — they didn't do or say the right thing, so you couldn't lose the weight.

Penny, from Houston, told about how she'd always wanted to lose weight to please her husband, who was commenting on how attractive this or that thin woman was. "I could never do it right or get thin enough for him," she said. "When I took the seminar, I realized that there was someone more important than he was. *Me.* I'd been so busy thinking about what *he* wanted, I'd never even thought about what *I* wanted. When I realized that I wanted to be thin just for myself, the pounds started rolling away very quickly!"

There's really only one person you have to please in life, and that's yourself. If you don't please yourself, the rest of it isn't worth much. You're still not happy. After I realized that I'd re-created my father's body and that I could now move on to creating my own, I didn't look around for the body I thought other people would like. I looked for the kind of body I would want to have if there were no one else on earth.

The body you create will be yours and yours alone. You might as well create it to please the person who will be inhabiting it and no one else. If you do it for your own reasons and in your own way, your motivation is going to be very strong indeed. Nothing will get in your way.

Let the vision of your new body flow out of you as naturally as the air you breathe. Let it be all yours, a tribute to how much you love and value yourself. You're not doing it because you have to, or because you're bad if you don't, but because you want to. You're going *toward* something, rather than running away from something.

Your breakthrough is going to look different from anyone else's. It has to, because it's uniquely yours. For some people it's like fireworks going off. For others it's like a quiet remembering. Some people can recall the exact moment it happened, and others only know that something has changed. Let yours be the way it is, without any judgment or criticism. That's exactly the way it's supposed to be. The important thing is that you're doing it for yourself, and not for anyone else. That way it will last, and you can enjoy all the richness of it.

EXERCISES (10 minutes)

1. List the people for whom you've tried to lose weight for in the past.

a.

b.

c.

d.

e.

2. "These are the reasons I want to lose weight for myself now:"

a.

b.

c.

d.

e.

A Gift To Yourself

What if the magician Merlin appeared to you and said, "I have a gift here for you. It's a thin body and peace of mind. If you take it, you'll never have to agonize about your weight again." Would you take it?

That's not just a fantasy. That same experience is available to you, except that you have to play the part of Merlin. You have to be just as generous with yourself as he would be, just as willing to give it to yourself, and just as sure of your power to make it happen.

You don't think twice about giving presents to other people. But when was the last time you gave yourself a gift just because you were you? There doesn't have to be a reason, and it doesn't have to be expensive. It can be a walk in the middle of the afternoon, a bubble bath, notepaper, a single flower. It doesn't matter what the gift is. What matters is the thought behind it, the fact that you cared enough to do something nice for yourself.

That may not sound like much, but giving yourself little presents and little doses of positive attention is like training for the big gift — a thin body. You're giving yourself the gift of you.

EXERCISES (5 minutes)

1. Have you ever given yourself a gift? If yes, how did you feel when you did it?

2. Name one thing you might give yourself, and tell how you would feel about receiving it.

Committing Yourself to Being Happy

Very few people would say or tell us that they don't want to be happy. Most of us would do almost anything to be happier than we are now. So why doesn't it always work? Why isn't everybody happy?

The problem is that most people think that happiness is something they're moving toward, which is always over there somewhere. They think that when they do or have certain things, then they'll be happy.

They go through four years of college thinking, "When I graduate, I'll have it made." When they get out, though, how long does that happiness and satisfaction last? All right, they've graduated, but now they have to get a job before they can be really happy. So they get a job, but then they think they'll be even happier when they get a raise.

It's the same with a vacation. They plan it all out, budget the money, look at the wonderful posters of people lying on the beach, and think, "When vacation time comes and I'm lying on the beach in Hawaii, then I'll be happy." But they get there, and it's not like the travel posters. They ask themselves where all the fun is. "Maybe it'll be tonight at the luau. Maybe tomorrow on the tour of the volcanos." They spend their whole lives waiting for it to happen to them.

They withhold complete happiness from themselves until they reach the next goal, but as soon as they reach it, that goal disappears and there's another one out there. They're always trying to get from here to there.

Suppose point 1 is "here" and point 2 is "there." You're going from here to there, so you travel along the line until you reach point 2. But once you've arrived at point 2, it becomes here and point 3

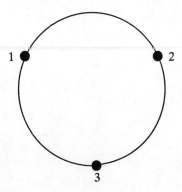

becomes there. So you start moving again, thinking that when you reach point 3 you'll be there. But as soon as you reach it, point 3 becomes here. That's one reason why people never get there.

If each of the points were a goal and the line were your life, what would it make sense to do? It seems like the only way to experience happiness is to put happiness where the line is, rather than where the points are. That way you would enjoy life all the time and still keep moving toward your goals.

The people who carry happiness with them wherever they go know that it's the trip, and not the destination, that matters. If you're taking a two-hour trip in the car to visit friends, is there any point in withholding your enjoyment until you reach your friends' house? You might as well enjoy the drive in the car, too.

In Aspen, Vivian said, "My breakthrough came when I realized I could go on like this forever, never letting myself be happy. I saw that after I was thin, I'd want new clothes, then a relationship, and so on. It was always going to be the same. There would always be something else out there. 'There's no end to this road,' I thought. 'When am I going to start enjoying it?' Now seemed like as good a time as any."

Happy people don't get that way by being lucky. They get that way by being committed to happiness. It's the most important thing in their lives. They know they won't be able to contribute much to themselves, to other people, or to the world unless they're happy. They keep in mind that it's possible to enjoy here just as much as there. They don't have to prove anything, and they don't need a reason to be happy. They just let themselves have happiness as a gift.

The commitment to being happy is a lot like the commitment to being a thin person. Both come from within you and arise out of a state of mind, rather than out of situations that are outside you. They both require permission to enjoy life and some generosity from yourself to yourself.

Sometimes children won't let themselves eat the icing until they've finished all the cake. They call it saving the best for last. That's a nice game to play with cake, but you cheat yourself if you play it with life. Not letting yourself enjoy living as a thin person until you've proven that you can take the pounds off is a sure way to keep them on. Bringing your thinness along with you every step of the way and enjoying it now are sure ways to win.

I have a friend who always used to say, "What are you waiting for, the Junior Prom?" The only reason to keep your happiness and your thin person on hold until after you've lost weight is that you don't think you deserve them, and that's the very foundation of theDiet Mentality. We've already seen how well that works. Let yourself deserve them now, even if it's against your better judgment, and see what happens. You may get to have your cake and eat it, too.

EXERCISES (15 minutes)

1. Are you committed to being happy? If yes, describe your commitment.

2. If no, what would it take for you to make that commitment?

a.

b.

c.

d.

e.

3. Write down the name of someone in your life whom you have loved unconditionally, exactly the way they are. Could you love yourself right now, in this body, the same way you love that person? How would you treat yourself if you could?

CHAPTER 10

The Physical Transition

Well, here you are. What do you do now? It's a little like being set down on a strange planet. You don't know how to act. You don't know where anything is. It's an exciting new world, but what do you do next?

First of all, give yourself a little time to make the transition. You've begun a whole new life, and you want to be gentle with yourself. Don't expect to wake up the first morning knowing everything you need to know to be a thin person. When a baby first learns to walk, he doesn't go out the next day and try to break the record for the hundred-meter dash. This is a time of transition, a time when you're in the process of moving from being a fat person to being a thin person. Sometimes it takes a while, so be patient with yourself.

As I was making the physical transition, I discovered several things, several principles or techniques, that supported the thin person and made it easier for him to emerge.

Levels of Hunger

Thin people eat when they're hungry and stop when their body has had enough. As we discussed in "Thin For a Day," you'll need to be clear about when you're hungry and when you're not.

The following is an expanded explanation of the hunger scale:

1. You're wobbly and dizzy. You can hardly think. The gas gauge isn't nearing empty, the car has already stopped. There's absolutely nothing in there. Most people have to go at least a day without food to get close to a 1.

2. You're still very hungry, but you could probably stagger to the dinner table.

3. You could definitely eat, but you're not on the verge of collapse.

4. You're starting to get a little hungry. Your body is starting to send messages that you might want to eat.

4.9. Your body has almost had enough.

5. You aren't hungry any more. Your body has had what it needs and is satisfied. This is where thin people stop eating.

5.1. You've put more food into your body than it needs.

6. You're a little full, but you could eat more. You could force down another helping, even though your body no longer wants anything.

7. You're becoming uncomfortable. You're starting to feel as if your stomach has stretched a few inches. The bloat is starting to creep up on you.

8. You're more than full, and it's starting to hurt. You almost wish you hadn't had that second helping.

9. Your body is screaming, "Get me out of here!" and the pain is setting in. It's absolutely no fun anymore. You feel as if they're going to have to put you on a truck and haul you away.

10. This is Thanksgiving Day full, when you have to roll yourself to the couch after dinner and all you can do is sleep. You didn't realize you were eating that much, and now you wish they would cut it out of you. You hurt for hours and swear you won't eat for a week.

If your hunger level is under five, you're feeding your body. If it's over five, you're feeding your head. Only it's your body, not your head, that gets fat.

When people first start to work with the levels of hunger, they get confused. If you haven't ever really experienced hunger and you feel the slightest twinge in your stomach, you may think you're at a 1 or even a 0. Actually you're probably closer to a 3 or a 4. Figuring out your level of hunger takes a little time and practice.

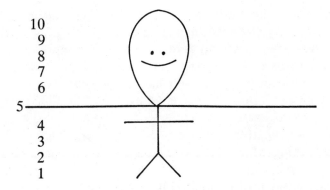

First close your eyes. Then place your hands on your stomach and ask your body if it's hungry. Is it a 4? a 3½? a 6? Listen to what your body says. It can give you a lot of information if you learn its language. You may not have talked to it in quite a while except to berate it, so it may be shy. Listen again. It will tell you. The more you listen to it, the more it will have to say.

EXERCISES (1 minute)

1. What is your level of hunger right now?

2. What would you guess is usually your level of hunger when you eat?

Only the Best for the Kid

The second principle of Diets Don't Work is to eat exactly what you want. Thin people feel that if they're going to all the trouble to eat something, it should be something they really like to eat.

If you've been on lots of diets, you've been programmed to ignore what it is you like and trained to eat dozens of foods you don't like. The whole idea of choosing food that is absolutely delicious may be scary or unimaginable to you. Janet, from Houston, told me that after taking the seminar she found grocery shopping an entirely new experience: "The first time I went shopping after taking the seminar, I realized that I had programmed myself not to even look at certain shelves in the store. I kept having to stop and back up, because I'd find myself whisking by whole aisles of food that had previously been off limits. It took me a number of weeks to reorient myself so that I felt like anything and everything in the grocery store was available for me."

Almost everyone who takes our seminars reports that they're amazed to discover they haven't really tasted the food they've been eating. Discovering what you like, what your 9s and 10s are, is really an adventure. Again, it's a matter of looking inside rather than outside yourself for clues to what to eat.

As you begin to choose foods that are 9s and 10s, you'll discover a funny thing. Many foods will remain a 10 for only a short period of time; their big attraction was that they were forbidden. Once you get enough of them, you'll find yourself wanting them only occasionally.

Another thing you can expect is that your body is going to want to eat funny things at funny times. For instance, I got up one morning and asked my body what it wanted for breakfast. The dialogue went something like this:

> Me: What do you want for breakfast this morning?
> Body: Rocky Road ice cream from Baskin-Robbins.
> Me: Come on. Are you crazy? Stop kidding around. What do you really want for breakfast?
> Body: Rocky Road ice cream.
> Me: Look, you don't understand. We're talking breakfast — eggs, bacon, toast, orange juice, cereal, stuff like that. Come on, what do you want?
> Body: Rocky Road ice cream!
> Me: You're crazy, I'm not listening to you anymore.

So I ate bacon, eggs, and toast for breakfast. The only problem was that I wasn't satisfied afterward. My body still wanted Rocky Road ice cream. The next morning when I asked my body what it wanted, this is the dialogue that ensued:

> Me: What do you want for breakfast this morning?
> Body: Rocky Road ice cream.
> Me: OK, but Baskin-Robbins doesn't open until 11:00 A.M., you're going to have to wait till then.
> Body: Fine. I'll wait.

So at 11:00 a.m. I was waiting outside Baskin-Robbins with my nose pressed up against the glass. I bought my scoop of Rocky Road ice cream, ate it, and was totally satisfied. I didn't eat again until 6:00 p.m. That's all my body wanted.

The first time, I listened to the voice of outer-centered reality: "Nobody eats ice cream for breakfast." The second time, I listened to my body, to my inner self, and I was satisfied. Do you begin to see the difference? You could just as easily find yourself wanting to eat breakfast foods at lunch or dinner. For example: "What do you want for dinner? A bowl of cereal with strawberries? Great!" You see, there really are no rules, and if you watch naturally thin people, you'll see this principle at work.

The Rule of Three

What if you're halfway through a meal, and you can't tell whether you're full or not? Stop and ask your body if it's had enough food for now. Constantly stay in touch with your body, especially when you're eating, and listen to what it's telling you. When you get to a 5, stop.

But when you're in the middle of a meal, it's sometimes hard to tell where you are. That's when you use the *rule of three*. The rule of three simply means that if you don't know whether you're hungry or not, give yourself permission to have three more bites. Not just any three bites, but the three most delicious bites on the plate. Go for your favorites. Eat the foods that are most appealing. Then ask your body again. If you're not getting any signals, the chances are that you've passed 5 and are feeding your reasons for eating, rather than your body.

Conscious Eating

Remember the story of how most of us eat popcorn at the movies? We really enjoy the first two bites, and the next thing we know there are nothing but seeds left at the bottom of the box. That's unconscious eating — you don't taste or enjoy the food. Your hand goes from the plate to your mouth and back again of its own accord. You've become an automatic eating machine.

What if you were very careful about what you ate each day, and then every night a demon slipped into your room after you were asleep and poured food down your throat. You wouldn't think that was very funny, but that's exactly what you do when you eat unconsciously. If you're going to eat, savor and appreciate it as much as you can.

Greg, from Pleasant Hill, California, tells this story about his first conscious meal after the seminar:

"I gathered together all my favorite foods and was planning on sitting down to the best meal of my life. I had a nice big New York steak, some green beans with slivered almonds, and a baked potato. I put it all out on the table with nice china and glassware, and I didn't do any of the other things I usually do when I eat. No TV, no magazines. I just ate. I cut into the steak and really savored it. Then I tried a couple of the green beans and they were delicious. Everything was great, but it seemed that it was taking an awfully long time to eat, and I was already starting to get full. About five minutes later I was stuffed. And I had only eaten half the things on my plate!"

Food is very different when it's eaten consciously. When you're aware of what you're putting into your mouth and enjoying it, you don't need to eat nearly as much. You don't want to. You're experiencing eating, rather than just shoveling food through a hole in your face.

I've found two things that helped me break the transition from unconscious to conscious eating. The first is to disconnect the eating machine, which we discussed in "Thin for a Day" — put your fork down *before* starting to chew. The other thing I discovered is to stop halfway through the meal, put my fork down, and stop eating completely. Then I take a moment to think about what I'm going to do after the meal is over. Otherwise I find that I can go on eating forever.

EXERCISES (1 minute)

1. "These are the activities I engage in and the things I think about when I eat:"

a.

b.

c.

2. Next time you get hungry, gather together the ingredients for a particularly enjoyable meal, and eat the meal consciously. Look at the food. Smell it. Touch it. Taste it.

Starving is Out

Sometimes when people start to think thin, they overdo it. The feeling of actually being hungry is so new to them and makes them so high that they want to do it all the time. They go for days without eating, just trying to see how hungry and high they can get.

The problem with letting yourself get too hungry is that, in the end, there is a tendency to binge. You're so hungry that when you finally do eat, you think you're never going to stop. Not only that, but you feel as if you deserve to eat two days worth of food at one sitting. Again, it doesn't work because it hooks you back into the Diet Mentality. Food becomes a reward that you have or haven't earned.

Starving and then going on a binge defeats the purpose of thinking like a thin person. It puts emphasis on food or the lack of it. One way or another it makes food important. One of the underlying principles of thinking like a thin person is that food isn't all that significant. You eat it when you're hungry, enjoy it, and stop when you're full. If you're alternately starving yourself and then going on a binge, your life is still centered around food.

EXERCISE (3 minutes)

"These are the ways I've felt, physically and emotionally, when I've starved and binged in the past:"

a.

b.

c.

d.

e.

Mastering the Clock

You don't have to eat just because it's a certain time of day, either. Meal times are set up arbitrarily. People in different parts of the world eat at different times of the day, and there's nothing sacred or particularly natural about breakfast, lunch, and dinner.

It might be interesting if just for a week you ate only when you were hungry, as if breakfast, lunch, and dinner didn't exist. When do you suppose you would be hungry? It would probably be different for you than it would be for another person. People get hungry at different times and in different ways. There's such a thing as the cocktail hour, but you already know that you don't have to have a drink every evening at 6:00.

Eating by the clock is a good way to fall back into unconscious eating. The clock says noon, so you start putting food into your mouth just because the hands on the clock are pointing up. You don't think about whether you're hungry, or even about what you want to eat. You just move automatically toward food.

Eating because it's time to eat doesn't even have to center around breakfast, lunch, and dinner. You may have a friend with whom you always take your morning coffee break. Each day the two of you go down to the cafeteria or the deli and grab a bite to eat. You do it as a ritual, more out of habit and companionship than out of hunger. Ask yourself whether you want to continue doing that. You can still take breaks with your friend, but you can change the ritual. You might want to start ordering tea rather than a sweet roll. The important thing is that you don't have to continue doing something just because at one point it became a habit.

Another way you can use time to fool yourself into eating more than you want is by saying, "If I don't eat now, I'll be starving by the time dinner comes." Maybe you will and maybe you won't. Eat what you want now, and let later take care of itself. Your eating habits and patterns will be changing. You might not get hungry at the same times. Let your body develop its own patterns. Avoid preventive eating. Carry an apple around in your pocket if it makes you feel more secure.

And who said you had to wait till dinner to eat, anyway? You can eat anytime you're hungry, even in the middle of the afternoon. Don't get caught up in the arbitrary structure of meals. You and your body are in charge, not the clock.

EXERCISE (2 minutes)

"These are the ways I let the clock determine when and what I eat:"

a.

b.

c.

d.

e.

Hungry or Thirsty?

When I first started eating like a thin person, I discovered something that shocked me. I was in the habit of heading for the kitchen as soon as I sensed messages from my stomach or my mouth that said, "I want something!" Notice that they didn't say, "I'm hungry." They just wanted something. The rumblings were probably more in my head than in my stomach, but off I'd go to the kitchen.

After I started thinking like a thin person, I'd stop in the middle of the kitchen and ask myself, "At what level of hunger are you now?" Silence. There was no real hunger, just a craving for something.

Then I tried drinking water instead of taking food, and about 90% of the time, the craving would go away. As it turned out, I was thirsty, not hungry, but my mind had learned to interpret any kind of craving as a craving for food.

More and more often I found that a glass of water would satisfy my "hunger." Most of us don't drink as much water as we need.

If I was still hungry even after drinking the water, I'd have something to eat. But I'd put my hunger to the water test first.

EXERCISE (1 minute)

The next time you feel hungry, try drinking a glass of water and see if the "hunger" goes away.

About Exercise

Kids love to move their bodies. They don't even think of it as exercise, it's just something that feels good. They're attuned to their bodies just as animals are. You were a kid once, remember? Do you recall when you lost that joy in movement?

For most of us it was in school — we were trained to sit still. If we didn't, we risked a poor grade in conduct. After years of such training, we were able to sit for hours and hours without moving. Then came TV — more sitting. And when we gained our weight, we became even more of a spectator and less of a participant. It's time to reverse that downward spiral. It's predicted that by the year 1997, one-third of the people in this country will be walking, jogging, biking, or roller skating to work. If you live far from work, you'd better start getting in shape now.

Exercise should be a gift you give your body. Listen to your body, and it will tell you when it wants to move around and play. Do exercise that produces results for you and that you enjoy. If it's unpleasant and makes you miserable, then don't do it. Once you get into shape again, exercise will relax you, eliminate stress, and make you look younger and firmer.

Many people exercise as if they're punishing their body. When they work out at the spa or gym, it's almost as if they're saying, "Take that! and that!" They look grim and don't seem to be enjoying themselves at all. It doesn't have to be that way.

When people come to our Golden Venus Spas in California and Nevada, they're amazed at how much fun we make it for them. Of course, they're there to get results, but we want them to approach the weights and exercise machines with the same playful attitude that a child displays on a playground.

We've also found that we have to hold people back in the beginning. They have no idea how out of shape they are. It's better to do too little than too much at first. In fact, you can usually cut in half what you think you can do easily, and even that will be too much. Start very slowly. Risk being lazy. Just do a little today and a little more tomorrow. It takes six weeks to get in shape to start training at a high level. Is it any wonder that when you start out giving it all you have, you get sore and tired and want to quit?

Years ago the mother of one of my friends became overweight, then went on a crash diet and lost thirty pounds. The problem was that she didn't look much better than she did before she lost the weight. In those days it was assumed that you were either born with a well proportioned body or you weren't. Most people didn't know that they could sculpt their bodies to exactly the shape they wanted.

Behind every curve in your body is a muscle, and how firm and well toned that muscle is determines how nice that curve looks. An attractive, well shaped body is something that most people have to work for, but it shouldn't be painful. Exercising with weights and equipment is probably the fastest and surest way to get the shape you want.

A few words about jogging: it's great for people who are built for it. The problem is that if you're overweight, your body isn't designed to do this form of exercise very well. Also, even though your heart and lungs are strengthened, jogging doesn't produce the beautiful, sculptured look that lifting weights does. Most people don't realize that jogging three miles and walking three miles accomplish almost the same benefits. By walking, you burn the same amount of calories, don't have to spend a lot of time warming up, cooling down, and stretching out, don't need to buy elaborate jogging shoes, and can fit your exercise more easily into a busy schedule. Instead of having sit-down meetings with my associates, I take them for a walk when we have something to discuss. It adds a relaxed pace to our all-too-hectic lives.

In Europe people walk almost everywhere and often carry canes or walking sticks. When I tried one, I was amazed at how much more enjoyable it made walking. It helps keep your posture straight and tall and isn't a bad crime deterrent either. If everyone in our country began walking with walking sticks, we might end crime on the streets and keep in shape at the same time.

EXERCISES (15 minutes)

1. "These are the reasons I haven't exercised in the past:"

a.

b.

c.

d.

e.

2. "These are the ways I've punished my body with exercise in the past:"

a.

b.

c.

d.

e.

3. "If I chose to exercise, these are the things I would ao to enjoy it:"

a.

b.

c.

d.

e.

Trust Your Body's Instincts

Your body knows more than you may think it knows. It's not just some dumb package you wrap yourself in, feed, and drag around from place to place. It's a living entity, with its own way of doing things and its own special kind of knowledge. Think of all the things your body does without your awareness: your heart pumps, your food is digested, air is breathed and assimilated, millions of cells are manufactured and sustained, delicate chemicals are kept in balance, even when you're asleep.

The body's instinct is to keep itself healthy and to heal any part that's not well. If you cut your finger, your body rushes to heal the cut, closing the wound and providing a natural dressing. Every day the cut gets smaller until in a week or so you can't even see it. Even your bones mend themselves when they're broken.

Your body gravitates naturally toward a state of health and comfort and acts without thinking for self-preservation. But you can slow down the healing of the cut on your finger by picking at it, by interfering with the body's natural processes. In the same way, you can slow down or stop your body's natural progress toward a healthy weight by picking at it mentally. Feeding your head and your emotions rather than your body makes it harder for the body to do its job. It's crying for one thing and being told, "Shut up and eat this." It's not getting the kind of fuel it needs.

Left to its own devices, your body will find what it needs. If it needs more protein or more carbohydrates, it will crave foods that are high in protein or carbohydrates. Just like the woman who found herself craving parsley and raisins and then discovered her body was screaming for iron, you can begin to tune into your body's signals.

I once read of an experiment in which children suffering from malnutrition were put into a room filled with food. There were all kinds of delicious things to eat, including sweets and candy, and in the corner there was a kettle of gruel. The gruel wasn't nearly as appetizing as the rest of the food, but it was loaded with all the nutrients the children's bodies lacked. The children were told they could have anything they wanted, and almost without exception they headed for the gruel. They couldn't get enough of it. They didn't think about what they *should* eat, they just followed their bodies' instincts.

Food cravings are something you already know about. The next step is to be able to determine whether those cravings are coming from your body or from your head. If you've been depriving yourself of certain foods because you thought or were told you shouldn't eat them, you may crave those foods just as much as the foods your body needs. There are emotional cravings as well as physical cravings.

In a similar study one of the little boys in the room full of food didn't go for the gruel, he went for the Crackerjacks. For a week he ate Crackerjacks for breakfast, lunch, and dinner. By the seventh day that craving was satisfied, and he started eating other foods. And at the end of the month, the food he'd eaten turned out to be nutritionally equivalent to a balanced diet. You may go through a Crackerjack phase, too. But when you start thinking like a thin person and giving yourself permission to eat whatever you want, the Crackerjack phase will fade.

"I drank Coke," said Nancy in one of the Oakland followup sessions. "When I was a child, that was about the worst thing we could do. My mother had fits everytime we came home with one, and refused to keep them in the house. For five days I had a Coke in the morning, one with lunch, and a couple more in the evening. Then a strange thing happened. It was as if a voice inside me said, 'I'd really feel better if you didn't keep throwing so much Coke down here.' I tried to ignore it, but Coke just didn't taste good anymore, and I haven't wanted one since. I've simply lost my taste for Coke."

Fred, who took the seminar in San Francisco, said that in the thirty years he'd lived away from home, he'd hardly ever eaten vegetables. "I realized in the seminar," he said, "that my aversion to vegetables was just a way of rebelling against my mother, who always used to make me eat them. I decided that after thirty years I could stop doing that. I decided to forget every idea I'd ever had about what I liked and ask my body what it wanted. You know what it came up with? *Broccoli!* I hadn't had broccoli in a good thirty-two years, but it tasted delicious."

At this point you may be saying, "What do you mean, listen to my body? Is this some kind of code? My body doesn't talk!" Your body may not talk to you in words; sometimes it talks in feelings, hungers, and desires. If you listen to it and learn to speak its language, the messages will be clear.

At first you may be a little skeptical or embarrassed. You may go off to a corner and say, "All right, body, what do you want?" You listen and hear nothing.

"See?" you say, "My body doesn't talk to me. It doesn't even have a voice." Listen again. Your body isn't used to your listening to it. Communication may be a bit stilted at first, just as it is with a new friend. But if you listen patiently, knowing that you're going to get an answer, then your body will start coming out of its shell. In the beginning you might not want to demand a specific food from your body when you ask it what it wants. Instead, you might want to ask it what *kind* of food would taste good. Go for the substance of the food, the qualities it has.

Give your body a recipe. Does it want something hot or cold? Soft or hard? Salty or sweet? Bland or zippy? Solid or liquid?

You might ask your body, "What kind of food would taste really good right now?" And it might answer, "Something crunchy." You can take it from there, asking questions until you get the answer.

"French fries?" you ask.

"No. Too greasy."

"Carrots?"

"No. Too bland. I want something with some zip to it."

"How about an apple fritter?"

"Maybe, but it sounds pretty sweet."

"A plain apple?"

"Yes! That's it."

After a while you don't have to play twenty questions with your body. You just quiet down inside and ask, and it gives you the answer right away. The better listener you become, the more quickly you get your answers.

It's the same with exercise. Sometimes your body will want a lot of it, and sometimes all it will want is a nap. You can learn to listen to those things, too. Your body has a life of its own and knows exactly what it needs to sustain that life.

Thin people trust what their body tells them. They assume,

consciously or unconsciously, that their body knows what it's doing and won't steer them wrong. They let their appetite dictate what they eat and don't try to second-guess it.

They have the point of view that their body is their friend. They don't have to fight it. They can relax and let their body support them.

EXERCISES (5 minutes)

1. "These are the fears or concerns I have about trusting my body's instincts:"

a.

b.

c.

d.

e.

f.

g.

2. Are you willing at this moment to let go of those fears and trust your body unconditionally?

3. "These are the ways I would like my body to support me with its instincts:"

a.

b.

c.

CHAPTER 11

The Attitude Transition

We have discussed certain key things you need to watch out for and know in order to make the physical transition to thin. Similarly, there are several discoveries that will assist you in making the attitude adjustment to becoming a thin person.

The main thing is to be patient with yourself, give yourself plenty of time, and leave room for error. Expect things to be different — don't be surprised when people treat you differently, for instance. And keep your sense of humor. Remember, I've never met anyone who became thin by being grim and serious about it.

It's OK to Have Feelings

Most of the food habits we've talked about have an emotional dimension. They make you feel satisfied, or good, or bad. In most cases there's an element of emotional manipulation. In some cases the specific purpose is to get rid of emotions, to try to make them go away by literally stuffing them down with food.

Mixing food and emotions is a dangerous game, a game that's difficult to win. You're always going to have emotions, both positive and negative, and if you head for the refrigerator every time you start to feel a negative emotion, you're going to get very heavy in a hurry. If, on the other hand, you can unhook food from your emotions, you accomplish two very important things:

- Your weight is no longer dependent on how you feel;
- You can bring your emotions to the surface, experience them, and do something about them.

You can't deal with something you won't let yourself see. It's like playing Blind Man's Bluff. When you let emotions like sadness, loneliness, anger, and grief come to the surface and allow yourself to experience them honestly, you'll find that they dissipate of their own accord. Some people are afraid that if they let them up, those feelings will stay around forever, but just the opposite is true. We're changing, growing beings, and we're not going to stay stuck in any one state of mind too long.

Gail, who lives in Aspen, said, "The first week I couldn't believe it. I was crying all the time. One afternoon I realized that I was crying about my mother, who'd died the year before. I'd never let myself feel the grief then and had started stuffing it down with food. After a week the tears just stopped, and I feel better now than I have in the entire year since my mother passed away."

I sometimes put aside fifteen minutes when I can really get into some particular feeling — sadness or pity, for example. I may just sit down and make myself feel as sad as I can for fifteen minutes. When I'm finished, sadness is the last thing I feel.

Keeping your emotions down is like trying to hold back a dam. Sooner or later, if the pressure isn't released, the dam is going to break or overflow. And when it does, it will be far worse than the fifteen minutes you spent letting yourself feel those emotions.

We have emotional appetites as well as physical appetites, and those emotional appetites can't be satisfied with food. It's like trying to make a car run by putting water in the gas tank. It doesn't work. It's not the right fuel. Emotions, both positive and negative, are a healthy part of life. How would you know happiness without sadness? How would you know love without anger? They're all a part of you. To the extent that you can accept and experience them, you can go on to what's next. Trying to make them go away only allows them to torment you.

Ellen shared in the Oakland seminar, "Being assertive is hard for me. Rather than tell someone what I want, I'll swallow it. Literally." The problem didn't go away until she stopped putting food in her mouth to deal with her discomfort.

The side benefit, of course, is that you learn to handle your emotions quickly and easily, because if you let them come to the surface, you're no longer working in the dark. You can see what you're doing and deal with them truthfully and appropriately.

You can't feed alcohol to plants and expect them to be healthy. You can't put water in a car and expect it to run. You can't feed food to an emotional appetite and expect it to go away.

EXERCISES (7 minutes)

1. "These are the emotions I suspect I've been suffing down with food:"

a.

b.

c.

d.

e.

f.

g.

2. "These are the worst things that could happen if I let my emotions come to the surface:"

a.

b.

c.

d.

e.

Relating to Others as a Thin Person

When you first start living like a thin person, people are going to be surprised. They may also be upset. They may think you've gone completely bananas. When you order a pizza, they may look at you suspiciously and say, "I thought you were on a diet?" You can just turn to them and smile. "Yes. A Pizza diet." *Or better yet, tell them you're using the Diets Don't Work approach to losing weight.*

Most of them won't have read this book, so they won't know

what you're up to. Even when you explain, they may have some of the same doubts and concerns you did when you first considered living like a thin person. They may think you're going to balloon up to 600 pounds. They may think you've given up all hope of ever being attractive. They may think it won't work.

If you want to make it logical for them, you can explain the four steps.

1. Eat when you're hungry.
2. Eat exactly what your body wants.
3. Eat each bite consciously.
4. Stop when your body has had enough.

It's hard to argue with that. Anyone who eats like that is going to lose weight. It's just that they don't have to suffer in the process.

Some people think that anything worthwhile can be gained only through suffering and agony. They may find it hard to believe that your way can be so simple and easy and still produce results. Give it time. When they start to see the pounds and inches disappear, they'll believe.

Till then you just have to recognize that they're relating to you as the fat person they knew in the past, not the thin person you are now. You may have to establish a whole new relationship with them. Whenever you begin a new relationship with yourself, you have to start a new relationship with others, too.

The first thing you may want to do is to explain what you're doing. Realize that it may make sense to them, and it may not. Whether they understand it or not, you can still tell them what you want from them. They'll probably want to support you, but they may not know how. You have to tell them.

Erin, who lives in Los Angeles, shared that her husband used to take her out to romantic dinners twice a week, which showed that he really cared about her. But every time she was in a restaurant, something took possession of her, and she started to eat on automatic. Going out to restaurants wasn't supporting her in being the thin person she wanted to be. She told her husband she loved that he cared enough about her to take her out so often, but that until she got more established with herself as a thin person, she would rather have those romantic dinners at home. He understood, and he never would have known unless she told him.

Maybe you want people to praise you all the time for acting like a thin person. Maybe you want them just to shut up and leave you alone. Maybe you want to eat out all the time. Maybe you want to eat at home every night. Maybe you want them to read this book. Maybe you just don't want to discuss anything to do with weight for two months. It's up to you. There's no right way to do it. You have to look inside and see what will work for you and what ways of relating to them will support you best. You are the only one with the answers.

You may run into some resistance. People may think they know better than you do what's best for you. You have to ask yourself if that's the kind of person you want to have in your life. Sometimes it will be uncomfortable, but one thing is for sure — you'll find out who really supports you.

Have you ever noticed how some people are able to stay focused on what they want to do no matter what others may think of them? They just keep moving toward their goal, whether it be making money, losing weight, or becoming a good skier, and they enjoy themselves in the process. Everyone wants to be with such people, because it's a pleasure to be with someone who's having fun, confident in themselves and sure of what they're after. In the same way, if you concentrate wholeheartedly on living and eating like a thin person, you'll probably have a lot of people rushing to your support.

EXERCISES (10 minutes)

1. "These are the types of resistance I may encounter from the people in my life when I start living like a thin person:"

a.

b.

c.

d.

e.

f.

g.

h.

2. "This is how I will handle each of those types of resistance:"

a.

b.

c.

3. "This is how I want my relationships with other people to be when I start living like a thin person. This is how I want them to support me:"

a.

b.

c.

Goodbye, Deprivation

You automatically want to eat more of anything you don't think you can have. If you make certain foods off limits to yourself, it will only make them more tantalizing. If you say to yourself, "No more apple fritters. No more Oreos. No more sour cream on the baked potato," your mind will become preoccupied with just those things. You'll be playing right back into the Diet Mentality, setting up rules for yourself that can only have one of two results:

• You eat them anyway and feel guilty;

• You don't eat them, but life isn't worth living. You're a martyr, nailed to the cross. You go around with this huge burden on your shoulders, heaving enormous sighs.

That isn't what being a thin person is about. Being thin is about enjoying life more and ending your preoccupation with food. Part of the joy of living like a thin person is that you can eat whatever you want to. It's also one of the guidelines. If you're depriving yourself, you're thinking like a fat person, not like a thin person.

Your body is going to want certain foods, and it's going to go after them with a vengeance. Say your body tells you it wants asparagus with hollandaise sauce. "Hollandaise sauce!" you say. "You must be crazy. Do you know how many calories are in hollandaise? Why don't you have this nice lettuce leaf instead."

But if you eat the lettuce leaf, the little voice inside you will still be whispering, "Asparagus with hollandaise." So you say, "Here. If you have to be bad, eat this banana." You eat the banana, thinking surely that will shut up the voice, that if you stuff him full of food, he won't want anything, much less asparagus with hollandaise.

But you still hear the whisper. Finally, you get to the point where you just can't do without asparagus with hollandaise. You go to the kitchen and fix it, and finally your body smiles and relaxes. Now you have all the calories in the asparagus and hollandaise, plus all the calories in the lettuce and the banana. You would have been better off just eating the asparagus in the first place.

There may come a time when you *want* to make certain foods off limits. That's fine, but don't do it because you think you have to. Some people say, for instance, that every time they drink coffee, they feel terrible. The first time that happens, you don't want to moan, "Oh, no. I can never drink coffee again!" Give yourself permission to drink it a few more times. You will probably reach a point where you don't even want it. The pain you go through when you drink coffee, or whatever it is for you, will be worse than the pain of not having it. Your body will rebel against that food not because it shouldn't have it, but because it doesn't want it.

Your body's wants and needs may change, especially as the pounds start to go away. It may be that next week it'll be fine for you to drink coffee or eat the food your body didn't want last week. Stay attuned to your body, listening for the changes that are taking place.

And don't deprive yourself. Give your body what it wants. That's one of the hallmarks of eating like a thin person.

EXERCISE (5 minutes)

"These are the foods I've been depriving myself of:"

a.   e.

b.   f.

c.   g.

d.   h.

i.   r.

j.   s.

k.   t.

l.   u.

m.   v.

n.   w.

o.   x.

p.   y.

q.   z.

The Scale Can Be Your Enemy

You get up in the morning and step onto the scale. (You always weigh yourself in the morning because that way you haven't had a chance to eat in seven or eight hours.) One of three things has happened: you've gained weight, you've lost weight, or you've stayed the same.

If you've lost weight, you're ahead of the game and can afford to cheat a little. If you've gained weight, you may feel angry or depressed. If you've stayed the same, it looks as if what you're doing is for nothing. And what's the likely response to any of those three situations? To eat, of course. The scale can actually prompt you to eat.

The scale can work against you in other ways, too. Aside from the fact that it's very difficult to find a scale that's accurate all the time, using a scale can lead you to the misconception that how you look is determined by what you weigh. That's not always true.

The scale is one of the most inaccurate ways to measure fat loss that I know of. Your goal is to have your body look exactly the way you want it to, and the scale doesn't reflect that. If you want to use something to measure your progress, a tape measure is better than a scale. Or use your clothes. Pounds and inches are not the same. The scale may not say that you're losing weight, but if your clothes are getting looser, you know you're making progress.

A pound of fat is much larger than a pound of muscle, yet it takes fewer calories to sustain. In other words, the more fat you have in proportion to muscle, the fewer calories you'll need compared with someone the same weight. And the more muscular you are, the *more* calories you'll need. That's one reason you can watch someone who is thin and beautifully toned sit down and eat a huge meal without gaining weight. You can't figure out where they're putting it, but it's all going into their muscles.

Furthermore, after you get to be twenty-six years old, your body starts playing a trick on you. It takes half a pound of muscle each year and turns it into fat, whether you like it or not. It's called aging. With each year that goes by, another half a pound of what used to be muscle is now fat.

That's not so bad, you say, half a pound a year. But they add up. By the time you're thirty-six years old, you have five more pounds of fat on your body than you did when you were twenty-six, even if you weigh the same. The clothes that fit you then won't fit you now.

Have you ever had an old pair of slacks that are finally back in style and sent them to the cleaners expecting to be able to wear them again? But even though you still weigh the same, they no longer fit you. The cleaners seem to have shrunk them. But that's not what's happened. You just have five more pounds of fat than you did before, and it's bigger than the muscle it's replaced.

It's a cruel trick, but our bodies do that to us. And it's one of the many reasons scales aren't really the best way to measure your progress.

EXERCISE (3 minutes)

"This is what would happen if I didn't get on a scale for:"

a. A week:

b. A month:

c. A year:

Imaging

So how do you keep track of where you are? The best way I've found is to create a mental image of exactly the way I want to look and to work toward that. I keep that picture before my mind all the time and use it as a yardstick. There are several advantages to making such a mental picture.

First, it gives you a specific goal to work toward. You're not just losing weight for the sake of losing weight or for the vague purpose of getting thinner. You have a specific goal in mind. There's a wonderful poster that reads, "If you don't know where you're going, you're likely to wind up somewhere else." Creating a mental image of what you want to look like tells you exactly where you're going.

Second, you don't know exactly what you're going to find at the end of the rainbow. If you've been overweight for some time, you may not have any idea of what you're going to look like if you lose thirty pounds. That may, in fact, be much more than you want to lose, or much less. If you hold out the goal of thirty pounds, you may not know precisely where it will lead you. It's hard to tell exactly where those thirty pounds are going to come off. They may come off the places you least expect, and you'll find that in order to get where you want to be, you'll have to lose more. Or less.

Third, having that mental picture lets you use another technique that people have found very successful. It's called imaging. You create in your mind the perfect picture of whatever it is you want — a body, a car, a house, a job, a relationship. You have to be very specific, painting the picture in your mind down to the last detail. Then you sit back and think about it, enjoy it, and feel whatever emotions surround it. If you recreate it every day, an image as precise as that has a good chance of becoming a reality.

If you were exactly where you wanted to be right now, and you took off all your clothes and stood in front of a mirror and saw your perfect body, would you recognize it? If you don't have a clear, vivid picture of what it would look like, take some time to create one. Then you will know exactly where you're going and will have some additional help in getting there.

EXERCISES (5 minutes)

1. Close your eyes and recall the perfect body you created in an earlier exercise. Is that still exactly the body you want to have? If so, write the description again. If not, write the new description.

2. Repeat this exercise once a day for a week.

Don't Try — Do!

If you want something, you have to make it happen. It bothers me when I ask someone to do something and they answer, "I'll try." I never know whether it's going to happen or not.

Saying you'll try to do something, rather than saying you *will* do it, indicates that you're not confident you can make it happen. You're starting out with a disadvantage.

There is no such thing as trying to live like a thin person. You either do it or you don't. If you're trying, you've put something or someone else in charge of whether or not you succeed.

In the Diets Don't Work Seminar, we use a demonstration I learned at *est* to illustrate the difference between trying and doing. There is a chair in front of the room, and I invite someone to try to pick it up. A volunteer comes up, puts his hands on the arms of the chair, lifts it off the ground, and smiles triumphantly. When I tell him that's not "trying," that's called picking up the chair, his smile fades.

Then he just puts his hands on the chair. I tell him, "No, that's not trying, that's called not picking it up."

Finally he gets wise. He puts his hands on the arms of the chair and starts struggling with it without moving it off the ground.

When you're trying, you can't be doing. To say you'll try to do something is to say that you'll engage it in a struggle, that you're willing to wrestle with it. It has nothing to do with whether it will actually happen or not. All trying does is give you an excuse in case you want to abandon the project for some reason.

In some circles "try" is a dirty word. When people hear it, they roll their eyes and assume the thing isn't going to happen. They don't trust people who use the word "try" to get anything done, because such people obviously don't trust themselves or really don't want to do it in the first place. People who try keep themselves stuck in the process of moving toward something, and if they're stuck there, they can never reach their goal. The process of trying and the process of completing are two different things.

The first question people ask when I say this is, "But how do I stop trying?" They are starting to hear all the fat person's old tapes:

"You can't do that."

"Hah! I've heard that before."

"You know you can't be trusted."

It's like a computer program that comes rolling out of your mind. The only way you can stop it is to reprogram the computer. Put in tapes that say, "I'm going to do it. I'm going to make it happen."

Say to yourself, "From this moment on I'm a thin person. I think like a thin person, feel like a thin person, and behave like a thin person."

Just let that change happen inside you, without going back and thinking or worrying about it. Allow yourself to be thin right now. If you look at it for a moment, you'll see that there's really very little else you can do. Being thin is more a statement of what you're being than a question of what you're doing. Sure you follow the four guidelines of being a thin person, but they come naturally out of the change that's taken place inside you.

You have to put all your eggs in one basket. You weaken your resolve if you start out saying, "Well, I'll try living like a thin person for a week and see how it goes." You leave yourself an out, an excuse for failing. If you say, "I'm a thin person, and I'm going to be that way no matter what happens," then you've made the choice. You've already become a thin person.

You're the one who has to make it happen. You're the only one who can. When you say, "I'll do it," rather than, "I'll try to do it," you burn your bridges behind you. There's nowhere to go except in the direction you've chosen. Just doing it can make you your strongest ally.

EXERCISES (6 minutes)

1. "These are the ways I've been trying, rather than doing, when it comes to my weight problem:"

a.

b.

c.

d.

e.

f.

g.

h.

2. "These are the things I need to do in order to stop trying and make it happen:"

a.

b.

c.

d.

e.

f.

g.

h.

Do It Passionately

Anything you do passionately becomes fun. It doesn't matter whether it's exercising, doing needlepoint, making love, or advancing in your career. If you're passionate about it, it's exciting and you're having a good time.

Some people think that passion is a random thing that goes with some things and not with others. That's just not true. You can be passionate about anything, even doing the dishes. All you have to remember is that you're the one in charge of whether you're passionate or not, and that whatever you do is going to be a lot more fun if you do it with passion.

Passion has less to do with the activity than with your state of mind. One person can't imagine getting excited about jogging, while another person can't get enough of it. That person lives and breathes jogging. Her eyes light up when she talks about it, as if it were the most wonderful thing in the world. Some people get passionate about politics, and others could care less. Some people are passionate about clothes, and others aren't. It's not the activity but how you approach it. It's a matter of making life exciting and playing for high stakes.

Try it out the next time you're faced with something you want to get done but don't particularly want to do. Doing the dishes is a good example. See if you can work up some passion for the project. Treat it as if it were the most important, exciting task in the world. Allow yourself to enjoy every minute of it; don't think about anything else. You may find that you have more fun doing those dishes than you had at any other time in the day.

How you look and feel about yourself is an issue that's probably more important to you than the dishes. If you inject the element of passion into living life as a thin person, it will make it all the more fun. It will turn the barriers and obstacles into exciting challenges that you revel in overcoming. You won't have to mope around worrying whether it's going to work or not. You'll be too busy having fun. You'll love thin instead of hating fat.

EXERCISES (5 minutes)

1. "These are the things in life that I already do passionately:"

a.

b.

c.

d.

e.

2. "These are the ways I can play the game of losing weight passionately:"

a.

b.

c.

d.

e.

The Only Real Change Comes From Within

We've all seen people who are trying to be something they're not. The illusion doesn't last long, and you can tell that those people aren't enjoying themselves. The real transformation from being a fat person to being a thin person lies not in what you do but in how you think about yourself.

There's a difference between people who have become real nonsmokers and people who are still smokers but aren't smoking. The first group have no desire for cigarettes. The second group want cigarettes, they just won't let themselves have them. That's no fun, and that's not the pattern we want to follow.

If you try to follow the four guidelines for eating like a thin person without really thinking of yourself as a thin person, you'll probably encounter a lot of resistance from yourself. Those four guidelines grow out of a state of mind. Without that state of mind, they become just a better form of dieting.

The most important quality of a thin person's state of mind is freedom. A thin person has the freedom to eat whatever he wants, and he also has the freedom not to eat. Either way, he's not struggling with himself. There's no recrimination or guilt. One choice is no better or worse than the other. Because he's free, all the compulsions are gone. He is truly in a position to choose when and how to eat.

It's all right with him if his weight fluctuates a pound or two. He knows he'll lose it, that his body will be drawn back to the weight he wants to be. He doesn't have to keep watch over himself, judging every bite he puts into his mouth. He knows he can trust himself and his body, and that gives him an enormous sense of peace.

That peace and self-acceptance take away all the fear and anxiety, which are the main emotional blocks to losing weight. They also make life a lot happier. You're free to be yourself.

Someone told me this story about a student in a Zen monastery. He came to the monastery wanting to get enlightened, and they put him to work sweeping the floors. For years he considered and pondered, trying to decipher all the hidden meanings, trying to figure out the real significance of sweeping the floors. Then one day he realized that sweeping the floors was just sweeping the floors, and at that moment he was enlightened.

Being a thin person is as easy as you make it. It isn't complicated or significant — it's just being thin.

EXERCISES (7 minutes)

1. List the five guidelines from this chapter that you think will be most valuable to you.

a.

b.

c.

d.

e.

2. Make up three new guidelines not mentioned in this chapter that will be helpful to you.

a.

b.

c.

3. "This is the dollar value I've created for myself so far in reading this book: $_____." Today's date:_____ .

4. Can you honestly say at this moment that you have chosen and are committed to live the rest of your life as a thin person?   Yes_____ No_____ Not yet_____

Thank you for doing these exercises. By this time only 12% of the people who started to read this book are left, and you're one of them. Congratulations! You've had more courage, commitment, and perseverance than 88% of the people who started. Take a moment now and acknowledge yourself.

CHAPTER 12

Where Do You Go From Here?

Keeping Your Sense of Humor — A Reminder

Kenny Rogers has a line in one of his songs that goes, "If you're going to play the game, you've got to learn to play it right." Learning the rules of weight loss, or of life for that matter, will help you keep your sense of humor. And the first rule is: *Life and everything in it is a game.* Of course, it upsets most people to hear that losing weight is a game. It didn't seem like a game when they got up this morning and tried to squeeze into their clothes. But the fact is, this is a game we're playing.

In order for an activity to be a game, it has to involve a notion of value, of relative importance. In our case, for example, being thin is more important than being fat. But why? Why is anything more important than anything else? The true answer is that nothing is more important than anything else except by agreement. And who has to agree to make something important to you? You do, of course. It doesn't make any difference what anyone else considers important unless you also agree.

Why is it that certain activities in life don't look like games? The answer here is that games have different degrees of consequences. Wars, for example, are games that have very serious consequences. When you've told the world that you're going to be thin, thrown away all your fat clothes, and bought all new thin clothes, you've upped the consequences. The problem with a game that has serious consequences is that we start to forget that it's a game and that *we* were the ones who made it important in the first place. If the consequences get too serious, we stop playing to win and begin playing to avoid losing. Even worse, we may begin playing as if we have to win, and that's no fun. At that point we become grim, lose our sense of humor, and become our own worst enemy.

When we forget that this is a game we've created, we forget the purpose of playing the game. The purpose of playing the game and the goal of the game must never be confused. You see, the goal of a game is to win, but the purpose of playing a game is to be happy, to experience feelings of aliveness, and to express ourselves fully. If we forget our purpose for starting this game in the first place, we may wind up winning the game at the expense of sacrificing our happiness, aliveness, and self-expression. You invented the goal. If you lose your health or happiness in the process, what have you gained?

The purpose for everything you do is to be happy, isn't it? So lighten up! Play all out, have fun, and remember your purpose.

Developing Inner-Centered Reality

What happens now? Let's say you've already worked through all the obstacles that were standing in your way, and you've firmly resolved to go out into the world and think like a thin person for the rest of your life. You accept and love yourself and know that it's only a matter of time before you get a thin body to match your thin thinking.

Then tomorrow you get up and the first person you see looks you up and down and says, "You know, my aunt was just as fat as you are, and she found this great diet. . ." What do you do? Punch him out and head for the deli?

No. You take a deep breath, remind yourself that you're a thin person, and smile. Then you either tell him what you're doing, or you pat him on the head and walk on. You don't have to argue with him or convince him. It doesn't matter what he thinks about your weight. He may roll his eyes and laugh when you tell him about the Diets Don't Work approach, but that's *his* problem. You know what you're doing, and that's all that matters.

You are going to get very skilled at handling people like that, and you're going to learn a lot about *inner-centered reality*. Inner-centered reality is when your reality is determined by what *you* think, rather than by what *other* people think. It doesn't mean you can't listen to other people and value their opinions, but in the end it's up to you.

There's a whole world out there that hasn't yet given up on diets. Deep down they know that diets don't work, but they're still hanging on, digging those fingernails into the rocks even though they're slipping. They don't want to be told it's as easy as it is. If they admitted that, they'd have to admit they'd been wrong all these years.

"I started to accept inner-centered reality," said Barbara in San Francisco, "when I realized that nobody out there knew any more than I did. If I was going to accept anybody's reality, it might as well be my own!"

There are also a lot of people who think you can't eat what you want and still lose weight. What they don't consider is that you're eating only when you're hungry and stopping when your body has had enough. Those people may give you a hard time. They won't understand that you're eating to fill your body and not your head because they're used to relating to you the way you were before. They'll look worried and shake their heads.

You just have to know that you're doing what works for you. Keep focused on what you're doing, keep to your inner-centered reality, and keep putting one foot in front of the other.

EXERCISES (30 minutes)

1. "These are the ways I've let other people dictate to me what was important and what I wanted:"

a.

b.

c.

d.

e.

2. "These are some of the things I *want* to do for myself rather than *should* do for myself:"

a.

b.

c.

d.

e.

3. "If my life were exactly the way I wanted it to be, this is how it would look:"

4. "This is how I would feel:"

5. "These would be my new goals:"

a.

b.

c.

d.

e.

f.

g.

h.

Breathing Space

You may want to give yourself a little breathing space, too. We've found that it takes about four weeks to break the old habits, another four weeks to get established in the new ones, and at least another four before they start to become automatic.

At some point during that first week, you may find yourself eating for your old reasons. Maybe you'll be watching *M*A*S*H*, and before you know it, you've eaten more than your body wanted. You may have reached a hunger level of 6 at the first commercial, but you're still eating when they roll the credits.

This is an important moment. The key to moving through it successfully is not to beat yourself up. Just tell the truth about what you did, recognize that you forgot about being a thin person, and be more aware of the potential danger the next time you sit down to watch *M*A*S*H*. You'll slip, I promise you. That's normal. The important thing is to pick yourself up, gently dust yourself off and re-establish your sense of being a thin person.

The pattern of three four-week cycles is just a guideline. It may take you one week or one day or nine months. Just remember not to be too hard on yourself — it may take longer than you think.

EXERCISES (6 minutes)

1. "These are the ways I might be inclined to beat myself up if I stop thinking like a thin person:"

a.

b.

c.

d.

e.

f.

g.

h.

2. "These are the antidotes, the things I will do to stop if I start to beat myself up:"

a.

b.

c.

d.

e.

f.

g.

h.

Start on Your Goals

One of the first exercises in this book was to make a list of the goals in life that you hadn't yet realized and a list of 100 incompletions. Set out to complete them all in the next ninety days. Of course, don't add to them as you go along. If you think of some new ones, make another list for when you've completed your first 100. Now would be a good time to start — you may get too busy to eat.

Some people keep weight around as a problem because a part of them is afraid that if that problem went away, they would have nothing to do. Starting to work on your goals is a reminder that that won't happen to you. There will be plenty to do, as you'll see when you start on your list.

Some of the goals you may not think you can possibly accomplish until you're thin. Those are the best ones to start on now. Doing them will force you to think of yourself as a thin person and reinforce your new points of view.

You will see again that becoming a thin person isn't just about losing weight. It's a way to live life. You can bring the same love and positive energy to your other goals as you do to being a thin person. When those goals start to happen and your life starts to be the way you want it to be, you'll be amazed at how quickly you'll lose interest in food.

EXERCISES (10 minutes)

1. What is the first goal you're going to work on? _____

   _____

2. What is the first thing you need to do to accomplish that goal?

   _____

3. When are you going to do it? _____

4. Make a game plan for thinking like a thin person. "When I wake up in the morning, I will . . ."

"At 9;00 A.M., I will..."

"At noon, I will..."

"At 6:00 P.M., I will..."

"At 9:00 P.M., I will..."

"Before I go to bed, I will..."

Falling In Love

There is only one person in the world you can be absolutely, positively sure you'll be living with for the rest of your life — yourself. Your relationship with everyone else on earth comes out of your relationship with yourself. To the extent that you love yourself and recognize the beauty within you, you'll love others and recognize the beauty in them.

Up to this point there's been a big obstacle in the way of your falling in love with yourself. You saw it every time you looked in the mirror. You may have judged and criticized yourself and found it hard to love the person you saw.

Now you have the means to replace that negative attention with positive attention. You have the tools to begin a new life and a new relationship with that person in the mirror whenever you choose. It may take some discipline, but it's a positive discipline rather than a negative one because you're facing rather than avoiding the real issue.

The discipline you'll need is nothing more than remembering to think of yourself as the person you want to be, the thin person inside you. That person already exists. He or she will be your lifelong companion just for the asking. There is no need for games, criticism, or sabotage. It can be a life and a relationship filled with support, love, and happiness.

There can be more joy, peace, and accomplishment in your life than you ever dreamed possible. You can end weight as a problem in your life forever — today.

It's a simple choice — to think like a thin person or to think like a fat person. All it takes is commitment, and permission from yourself to let yourself be whichever you choose. Then the struggle will be over. You won't ever have to worry about it again, and you can get on with the rest of your life. You can start to let the joy, peace, and sense of accomplishment you feel spread out into the rest of the world. And you can make the greatest contribution to yourself and to others that anyone has ever made — to be and love yourself.

EXERCISES (5 minutes)

1. "These are the ways I give myself permission to love myself exactly the way I am:"

a.

b.

c.

d.

e.

2. "This is the exact dollar value I've created for myself by reading this book: $ _____."

3. "This is how I would describe my commitment to living as a thin person at this moment:"

_____

_____

_____

_____

_____

_____

_____

Today's date:_____.

Epilogue

It's up to you now. The life you lead from now on, whether as a fat person or as a thin person, will be the one you create for yourself. You can go back and reread sections of this book for inspiration, but the rest is up to you.

Thank you for letting me share with you some of the things I've discovered about living like a thin person and making life a joy rather than a struggle. You and I have an opportunity to do something that will make a contribution to the world. You can come to know that you have the power to create your body and your life exactly the way you want them to be. And as you end weight as a problem in your life forever, you can begin to help others do the same.

Good luck, and be happy.

* * *

Before I leave you for now, there's one last acknowledgement I would like to make. He's been ignored for too long, and it's time that we give credit where credit is due. Before you enroll your friends in your "new" method of losing weight, have them look up the word "Fletcherism" in the dictionary. It's derived from the name of an American nutritionist, Horace Fletcher (1849-1919), and means "the practice of eating in small amounts and only when hungry and of chewing one's food thoroughly."

Do you have questions about the Diets Don't Work Seminars? Call (415)531-8494 in Oakland, California or (713)981-5667 in Houston, Texas, or write Diets Don't Work Seminars, 2000 Rosecrest Drive, Oakland, California 94602.

Time Schedule. All day seminars are held on weekends from 9:00 a.m. until 9:00 p.m. Please arrive by 8:30 a.m. to allow enough time to check in. Lunch and dinner furnished at approximately 1:15 p.m. and 6:00 p.m.

Do you want to share your results and insights with others? Future news stories will contain specific results obtained from those who follow the *Diets Don't Work* method. Write to Bob Schwartz, 1015 7th Street, Galveston, Texas, 77550.

Do you want to order copies of *Diets Don't Work* **for friends or customers?** Call 800-227-1152. Quantity discounts available on request.

There are fifteen million people on our planet dying each year as a result of starvation, and there are hundreds of millions of people who are overweight. Let's involve the people who eat too much in making sure that those who are starving to death have enough to eat. You can make a difference. Write:

The Hunger Project
604 William
Oakland, California
94612